I hope they know.....The Essential Handbook on Alzheimer's Disease and Care.

I hope they know....The Essential Handbook on Alzheimer's Disease and Care

by

Zoë A. Lewis, M.D. FACP

"I Hope They Know...The Essential Handbook on Alzheimer's Disease and Care," by Zoë A. Lewis, M.D. FACP. ISBN 978-1-60264-177-8.

Published 2008 by Virtualbookworm.com Publishing Inc., P.O. Box 9949, College Station, TX 77842, US. ©2008, Zoë A. Lewis. All rights reserved. No part of this publication may be reproduced, stored in a retrieval system, or transmitted in any form or by any means, electronic, mechanical, recording or otherwise, without the prior written permission of Zoë A. Lewis.

Manufactured in the United States of America.

Dedications

OUR NATURAL GIFTS LIKE flowers flourish when nurtured. To my family, loved ones and teachers, I give my heartfelt thanks and appreciation and offer this book to them in gratitude for their encouragement, knowledge and love.

To the generosity of strangers, without which many of us would struggle against circumstances easily overcome with the power of kindness, compassion and empathy.

To those that smile. Each day we have an opportunity to make choices. At least once in a day with as little as a smile or act of selflessness, we can create a moment of peace for ourselves and others.

In memory of Jim Haggerty — a one-in-a-million man.

Acknowledgements

I WOULD LIKE TO thank my contributing authors and poets, each of whom enthusiastically participated in this project. I am grateful for your dedication and support of my efforts to bring this essential information and guidance forward, especially Myron Weiner, M.D.

The Alzheimer's patients enrolled in the Program of All-Inclusive Care for the Elderly (PACE) in Miami-Dade County at the Miami Jewish Home and Hospital, an affiliate of Florida PACE Centers, Inc. These folks and their consenting family member generously offered their art work.

Amide Midy, Certified Therapeutic Recreation Specialist, and Karen Wells, Director, both of the Miami-Dade PACE Program at the Miami Jewish Home and Hospital, Miami, Florida.

Elizabeth Cockey, Master Art Therapist and her artist - clients at the Good Samaritan Nursing Center, Baltimore, Maryland.

Table of Contents

PART I
Introduction

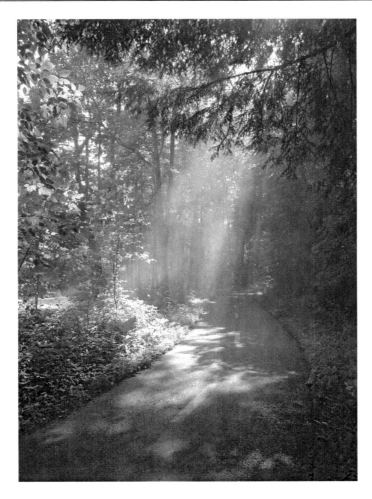

I BELIEVE LIFE IS a road. Along its course, long or short, we will come to understand our journey will hold surprises when least wanted, mysteries with no solution, even sadness, loneliness and doubt. But if we each strive to open our heart and keep it open even when the path seems darkest, we will always find joy, love, compassion and wonder in the miracle of being.

Z. Lewis

1

Preface

ALZHEIMER'S DISEASE IS A devastating world-wide problem. This disease alone will claim the lives of hundreds of thousands each year while it brings devastating emotional and economic burdens to the families of those afflicted. Alzheimer's disease now affects approximately 5 million Americans, and is currently the seventh leading cause of death in the USA. World-wide it ranks among the top ten causes of death. Unless a cure or prevention is found, it is estimated that the number of Americans with Alzheimer's will climb to 14 million by the middle of this century; between a third and a half of those over 85 may have Alzheimer's disease. The Alzheimer's Association estimates a new diagnosis is made every 72 seconds. Ongoing medical research and new models of care will change the course of this disease, but hope is the primary support for those with Alzheimer's disease today.

Preserving the quality and dignity of life as we become ill or approach death is my vocation. One of my most motivating and humbling moments occurred when I realized that despite my training in Internal Medicine, caring for Alzheimer's patients as their disease worsened presented unique challenges to my skills. I experienced new awareness, compassion, and most of all a sense of duty.

My change in attitude towards Alzheimer's disease occurred on the first day I entered one of the many long-term care facilities to which I had been assigned to care for patients with end-stage dementia. I came as a hospice doctor. I recall vividly how I began examining my first patient, my eyes focused on his absent stare as I listened to his breathing, almost synchronous with the gentle hum of his feeding tube pump. Suddenly, my attention was interrupted by a startled outburst from another patient's expressionless face across the room. At that moment as I looked around, everywhere I looked, I was overtaken by the despondent, eerie scene of vacuous expressionless eyes and slumped, effortless, motionless bodies. This scene repeated itself in room after room.

Bewildered, I asked myself how I had not already grasped the enormity of the situation.

At home that night I watched a World War II movie and finally cried. I remembered the patients. I realized then that some of them had been soldiers, and the women, the sacrificing wives of veterans. They were unaware because of their Alzheimer's disease that it was November 11, Veterans Day. What troubled me most was the thought that perhaps we were not doing our best for them, what Tom Brokaw has called *The Greatest Generation*. Were we helping them have the best possible quality of life they surely deserved after they had contributed so much to our lives and what we often take for granted, our freedom, our way of life? Or was it simply easier or the best solution to warehouse them and put them away in a safe facility and wait. Consider the fact that simply waiting, with or without dignity, is costing our government hundreds of millions of dollars annually for their care. The Alzheimer's Association predicts the costs will skyrocket to $400 billion by 2030, the size of the entire Medicare budget today. This disease will become a huge national problem that many are just beginning to grasp.

On Veterans Day years ago I recognized Alzheimer's disease for what it was—an undignified vector of death. It destroys the function of the mind, disables our human characteristics and deprives us of our ability to relate to each other. That Veterans Day marked my heart-felt commitment to improve the quality of life in end-of-life care. I challenged myself to imagine if there was a better way to deliver care with dignity and respect for the thousands of patients with this disease that was cost conservative as well. This book is dedicated to individuals with Alzheimer's disease and their families. Perhaps with greater guidance and education, families unaware of the existing resources for those with Alzheimer's disease can locate and use them, reducing the burden and suffering of many. Perhaps something as simple as a holding a paint-brush or a listening to a piano tune will improve their quality of life, even for moments.

About The Author

ZOË A. LEWIS, M.D., DAAHPM, FACP received her medical doctorate summa cum laude from the University Of Rome School of Medicine, 'La Sapienza', Rome, Italy. She completed her internal medicine residency training in the University of Pennsylvania Healthcare System, Philadelphia, Pennsylvania. She is board certified in Internal Medicine and Hospice and Palliative Medicine. She is a diplomat of the American Academy of Hospice and Palliative Medicine, (DAAHPM) and is a Fellow in the American College of Physicians, (FACP).

Dr. Lewis has worked with numerous hospices in Florida and most recently, in Boston, Massachusetts. She is the former Corporate Medical Director for Beacon Hospice, Inc. in New England and received specific acknowledgement for her leadership efforts by the National Hospice and Palliative Care Organization in their 2006 guide, Caring for Persons with Alzheimer's and Other Dementias, Guidelines for Hospice Providers. She is also the former Assistant Medical Director for the Caritas Good Samaritan Hospice also of Boston, and a former hospice team medical director for Vitas Healthcare in Broward County, Florida. Additionally, she led the initiative to implement the first hospital-based palliative care consultation service for St. Elizabeth's' Medical Center of the Caritas Christi Healthcare System in Boston. She was nominated for Fellowship into the American College of Physicians for her contributions to this clinical consultation service. Other achievements include a scholarship from Pennsylvania Hospital, Philadelphia, for elective study in Infectious Disease in Bangkok, Thailand.

As an internist in Boston, she provided primary care at Brigham and Women's Physician Group and for patients in the Caritas Christi Healthcare System. She held academic teaching positions at University of Pennsylvania, Tufts University Medical School, Brigham and Women's Hospital and Harvard School of Medicine. Active in both physician and community education on issues of end-of-life care and general medicine, she has regularly presented medical grand rounds in New England, South Florida, and nationally for hospice and end-of-life care conferences. She has numerous publications to her credit. She currently works as a consultant for hospice programs and continues to practice internal medicine. Her special interests are the development of art and music therapy programs for hospice patients with an emphasis on improving quality of life and compassion.

About The Contributing Authors

I HOPE THEY KNOW........is ultimately a self-help guide that discusses many areas of care. The contributing authors have generously added their experiences and knowledge to this book. I will share a few words why I chose these individuals and discuss their expertise with Alzheimer's patient's care and person-centered care. Their biographies are included at the end of this book.

Perhaps the most devastating crisis of Alzheimer's disease and the dementing illnesses is the gradual loss of the ability to communicate with others effectively as the disease progresses. Communication techniques that are nonverbal can be valuable resources in care. These techniques and care models can enable us to communicate without words, and restore our bonds and sense of connection with our loved ones.

Our prehistoric human ancestors, in what is now Lascaux, France, painted magnificent animals on the walls of caves more than 17,000 years ago. Creating figurative art is an intrinsic human medium of communication, and we begin to explore this nonverbal form of expression as children with our imaginations and elemental finger painting. Artistic creations are inspired from somewhere in the mind and we can express a wide range of emotions, even as the brain and its cellular components deteriorate. Alzheimer's patients retain their ability to express themselves artistically until late in the disease. Art is "in the moment". Together with published author, speaker and art therapist, Elizabeth Cockey, we guide you in the exploration of this medium as an expressive outlet and form of communication for Alzheimer's patients and their caregivers.

Music is another form of nonverbal communication. Most of us have learned some traditional childhood rhymes and later, the songs of our generation. More likely than not, over the course of our lives, we developed a growing appreciation of various music styles. Internationally recognized for her contributions to the field of music therapy and in particular her work with Alzheimer's patients, Dr. Suzanne Hanser of Berklee College of Music, Boston, explores the use of music to calm, comfort and stimulate an individual with a dementia illness.

Likewise using touch or gentle massage to elicit comfort and solace can be as effective as medication in producing a calming effect, while it enables a loved one or caretaker to show empathy. It can also be a form of nonverbal communication, and has been shown to benefit those with Alzheimer's disease at any stage. Gentle touch is one of many palliative medical care interventions. This kind of care-giving, also known as palliative care, is performed by a team of professionals, and is intended to promote and preserve quality of life and uses a wide range of techniques, practices, modalities and medical interventions. Observing and tracking response to those interventions is difficult in nonverbal patients. Without research to quantify interventions, we are left with empirical evidence or anecdotal evidence at best. Myron Weiner, M.D. describes his work with quality-of-life research and interventions with Alzheimer's patients. His research helped in my understanding of nonverbal communication, and provided the groundbreaking measures for patients with end-stage disease unable to communicate responses to interventions. His team of researchers developed an internationally used scale, the QUALID Scale that measures 11 behaviors that are thought to indicate quality of life. His contribution, "What is quality of life and where can it be found?" underscores the need for more research in this area. While we know that many of the newer treatment techniques cannot slow or reverse dementia, research evidence shows they can improve the quality of life for both a person with Alzheimer's disease and their caregivers. For this reason, I believe they are indispensable in Alzheimer's care.

My communication skills evolved with experience as an internist. I developed greater empathy and compassion from my hospice work as a hospice team physician. However, it was not until I lost a dear friend to cancer that I understood the pain, suffering and difficulties in expressing myself to him as a physician and friend. His loss also awakened new emotions and grief. It was following those first years of my career that I began to develop my approach to doctoring and communication skills that are nonjudgmental, compassionate and deliberate. I recognized people who are seriously ill, including a best friend, needed information about their disease in their language, with terms that they could understand. Debbi Dickinson will share her expertise and experience regarding the unique aspects of grief and bereavement with Alzheimer's disease and dementing illnesses. This illness presents challenges to loved ones like no other. Debbi's father suffered from Alzheimer's disease, and she shares her personal story.

True dialogue with patients enables them to process into their own lives and experiences what is happening to them. Physicians can never overestimate all of the emotional needs or the unique circumstances that affect the lives of our patients. We will not know what is best if we don't make ourselves available to ask and listen. Dr. Patricia Munhall, founder of The International Institute for Human Understanding, acclaimed author and practicing psychoanalyst will describe the emotional factors that evolve in loved ones as they lose the ability to communicate with a person affected by Alzheimer's disease.

No book dedicated to care giving would be complete without acknowledging the caregivers' needs as well as those of the patient. Self-awareness is fundamental in maintaining balance and wellbeing. I came to recognize caring for yourself while you care for others is not selfish. Each of us in life finds our own means to maintain our physical and spiritual heath in balance. I chose yoga and mediation. Kino MacGregor, founder of the Miami Life Center, is a world-recognized yoga instructor and a PhD student at New York University in holistic health. She shares her insight and knowledge into achieving the physical and spiritual balance with life's demands and struggles in the context of being a care provider. She explains why we need to honor our own care needs.

Fanny Barry, author, cancer survivor, and founder of That Barry Girl Foundation inspired me with her insight after her challenges with a deadly disease. Her books inspired mine. Her new-found approach to life and her dedication to public service and education were kindred desires as well. Her work is dedicated to inspire others overcome doubt, depression and survive during an illness. Her words and insight are uplifting for anyone struggling with a life-threatening disease.

Disease may destroy the body and the mind, yet reconnecting with our expressive side using the arts, through touch with gentle hands or any manner that allows us without the use of words to bond to each other, can somehow soften this mortal blow.

Alzheimer's Day Care and Wellness Programs

ADULT DAY CARE CENTERS and Wellness Programs throughout the country are resource centers for patients and families and can provide expert educational support and information beyond the scope of this book. I approached the Miami-Dade PACE program with the intent to observe their activities and especially to observe the interactions with clients in the art program. The art illustration and interpretation chapter is devoted to their work.

Directories for Day Programs in your area can be obtained from one of many national databases for Alzheimer's Care and Research, The National Alzheimer's Organization and The Program of All-Inclusive Care for the Elderly (PACE). Some day programs have state and or federal funding, while others are private pay. The National PACE Program provides a comprehensive range of medical and healthcare services for those who prefer to live at home and meet Medicare and Medicaid eligibility criteria.

Typical day programs are usually open from 9 a.m. until 3 p.m., Monday through Friday. Extended hours are often available in some locations. Transportation is usually included, and is typically provided by a van service or can be arranged at the facility. The range of activities is dedicated to helping people who are still living at home maintain physical and mental abilities. Participants are actively engaged in activities that maximize their abilities and promote a sense of accomplishment. There is usually a professional team of caregivers with good staffing ratios that assure individual attention and care. There is an interdisciplinary care team that is headed by a full-time program director and includes a nurse, social worker, activity director and program assistants. Medical, behavioral and dietary experts consult regularly in most cases. Each program with have unique individuals with their own strengths and weaknesses. People who work in these programs have usually received extensive education in caring for individuals with dementia illness and Alzheimer's disease. Behavioral interventions, communication techniques and appropriate activity programming are emphasized. Investigate the general schedule to determine if it is right for your circumstance. Each program has different strengths and incorporates local aspects, programmed into activities, but the best programs offer innovative ways to connect to community and offer family and caregiver support. After reading this book, you will be able to decide for yourself what kinds of services you think would best benefit your unique circumstances and be prepared to ask for help in achieving your care goals. There are numerous options you will come to recognize!

Part II
Early Diagnosis
Allows Prompt Intervention

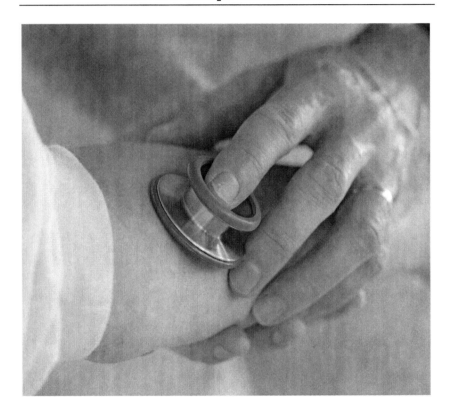

1
I hope they know....the facts.

EVERY 72 SECONDS SOMEONE is diagnosed with Alzheimer's disease.

Alzheimer's disease causes dementia. It is a neurological disease that affects the brain and the brain cells and was first described by a German psychiatrist, Alois Alzheimer in 1906.

More than 5 million people in the USA alone have the disease and it is the 10th cause of death world-wide. The disease progresses slowly over years or in some cases more rapidly and ultimately leaves the patient without the ability to recognize family or friends, eat, walk or simply smile. The simple things a child has learned, a patient with Alzheimer's will forget. Many times personality changes are so severe that family must resign the care to others for the patient's safety and protection.

The cause of Alzheimer's is not yet known and there is a worldwide effort under way to find better ways to treat the disease, delay its onset, or prevent it from developing. Age is the main known risk factor. Drug therapy can be successful in slowing down the process, and stabilizing memory, but early diagnosis is the key to the best outcome.

There are many features of Alzheimer's disease and it may seem complicated to appreciate the difference between other kinds of dementia illness and Alzheimer's disease. Treatments are different as well.

The first step should be recognizing the signs and symptoms. Once the diagnosis of Alzheimer's disease or another kind of dementia illness is made, then understanding, gathering information and support for the patient and the family can occur with the best care practices put into place. Many people joke about the declining mental acuity and memory challenges of the elderly, inferring certain behaviors are characteristics of advanced age, but Alzheimer's disease or any other form of dementia is a serious medical illness.

2
I hope they know....signs and symptoms of Alzheimer's disease and other dementias.

WE ALL HAVE HAD moments of confusion, trouble with organizing and expressing thoughts, misplacing things, getting lost in unfamiliar places, and changes in our personality and behavior when we are out of sorts or in a bad mood. Most people assume forgetfulness and memory changes are part of aging. Many assume the personality changes of the elderly stem from the resignation of old age and other kinds of debility from coexisting illnesses.

Progressive change in appetite, withdrawal from normal pleasures, change in intimacy and excessive sleeping, or chronic confusion can all be signs of many things, but also any of these signs may be an early symptom of Alzheimer's disease. Short-term memory problems are the hallmark, but they are not the only symptom. We accept that our bodies will age, but we fear memory loss. Just what kind of memory loss is associated with Alzheimer's disease and what is the kind that is a normal part of aging? *Procedural memory*, the memory associated with tasks such as how-to-eat, how-to-drive-a-car, how-to-tie-a knot kind of memory is the strongest type of memory. It is only affected by Alzheimer's disease in the later stages. Our *semantic memory* covers facts, like what is a spoon, where did I leave my keys, what is a key, and who was in the movie I just watched? This is the memory that is affected both in the aging brain and in early illnesses that lead to dementia, such as Alzheimer's disease. It takes longer to retrieve the information we store in the brain but the information remains in the normally aging brain. We can still learn, but it takes longer. For the Alzheimer's patient, both the ability to hold on to new information and the ability to learn new things are compromised.

The most characteristic symptom of Alzheimer's disease is a profound impairment of recent memory. This is seen as individuals begin to misplace everyday items, such as the car keys or eyeglasses routinely. They become disoriented and get lost in familiar surroundings, such as when driving on well-known streets. They often forget what they were doing in the middle of doing it.

Alzheimer's disease is the most common cause of dementia. Although not a difficult diagnosis for experienced physicians, the diagnosis is only 85-90% accurate and is only absolutely confirmed by brain biopsy after death.

Other causes of dementia must be considered and eliminated before the diagnosis of Alzheimer's is made. If you know someone who has these symptoms encourage them to see their doctor. There is no shame in being ill.

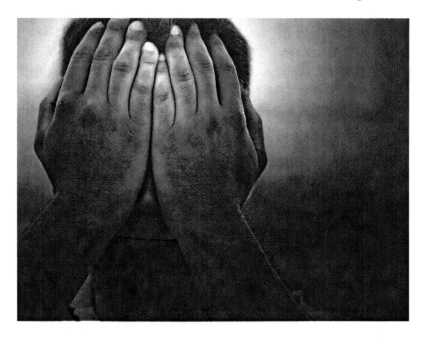

3
I hope they know....other causes of dementing illnesses.

THE TERM *DEMENTIA* REFERS to a disabling loss of the brain's ability to process information and communicate. Many diseases can cause dementia. Most are irreversible, but some are both treatable and reversible, so it is imperative that a doctor make the diagnosis as early as warning signs and symptoms of memory and behavior changes arise.

Treatable causes of dementia include normal pressure hydrocephalus, a condition caused by an increase of cerebrospinal fluid in the cavities (ventricles) of the brain, brain tumors, metabolic causes from other diseases like uncontrolled diabetes, thyroid conditions, low vitamin B12 levels, some simple or severe infections, including meningitis, medications, the inappropriate use of some medications, schizophrenia, severe depression, toxins, recreational drugs, alcohol, heavy metals, and industrial pollutants. This is a partial list, but a good history and physical examination by your doctor will include a thorough evaluation of all of the medications and recent changes in health.

The causes of nonreversible dementia include recurrent small strokes or large single strokes. This type of dementia, called *vascular dementia*, is the second most common form of dementia in the United States and Europe. Other diseases are Lewy body dementia, Frontotemporal dementia (which includes Pick's disease), brain damage due to prolonged low level oxygen to the brain as occurs with severe heart attacks, drowning or choking. Dementia can also occur with progressive supranuclear palsy, Creutzfeld-Jakob Disease, Parkinson's disease, Huntington's Disease and infections of the brain and its coverings, including syphilis and infections that occur in persons with immunodeficiency, such as AIDS.

4
My Father's Remains

My father's remains
still perceive,
still breathe.
Pursued by imaginings
through fantastic domains.

He defied fate
educated himself,
became an aviator,
kept his wife
from a wheelchair'd state,
endured her soundless
compassion-less world,
fought to maintain dignity
and autonomy,
but lost, woefully.

I cry; not for me, but
who he used to be;
confident,
arrogant.
Now, only living flesh — without
dignity, or direction
or pride.

Wanting it over,
groping for an exit
from the pain, but
his remains... remain.

Myron Weiner, M.D., © 2000

5
I hope they know....how the disease can be diagnosed.

YOUR DOCTOR WILL WANT to do some simple blood tests that can reveal other causes for the change in memory and changes in behavior. These are standard and any doctor can perform them. Other diseases that cause dementia-like symptoms may be discovered with a simple physical examination and laboratory tests. A visit to your doctor is the first step in discovering the diagnosis.

Standard lab tests for Alzheimer's disease include:

Complete Blood Count (CBC)
Thyroid panel: T3, T4, TSH
Liver function tests (LFT)
STD testing: VRDL for syphilis, HIV test
Vitamin B12 and folate levels
Brain imaging with CAT or MRI scans
Calcium and other electrolytes
Kidney function test

The list is relatively short for the initial work up and many of these tests are standard tests. Some are the blood tests done in yearly physicals at the time of check ups along with blood pressure monitoring, diabetes screening and other preventative care measures. The second round of testing is more focused and may be done by a neurologist, geriatrician or other specialist like psychiatrists that specialize in behavior and memory disorders.

6

I hope they know....several alternative tests may be helpful.

NEUROLOGISTS, GERIATRIC PSYCHIATRISTS AND geriatricians are also medical doctors most likely to perform more specialized tests if there is some doubt about the cause of symptoms. The most common include:

Tests of brain function such as neuropsychological testing SPECT and PET scans

Less common but occasionally used:
Homocysteine levels
Hair mineral analysis to assess heavy metal toxicity (aluminum, arsenic, mercury)
Lyme test and other tests that evaluate infectious diseases

Not usually performed but mentioned by some researchers, these blood tests include:

A comprehensive hormone panel, including estrogen (E1, E2, and E3), progesterone, testosterone, and melatonin
Adrenal function test, including cortisol and DHEA
Oxidative stress levels
Essential Fatty Acid Panel
Markers of inflammation, including C—Reactive Protein (CRP)

7

I hope they know....what we currently understand about the cause of Alzheimer's disease.

THE CAUSE OF ALZHEIMER'S disease is unclear. Several mechanisms have been proposed. A world-wide effort in research is ongoing. The mechanism currently thought to begin the disease process is the accumulation in the brain of a protein called beta amyloid, due to overproduction of the protein or inability of the brain to remove it. The accumulated beta amyloid is deposited in the brain in microscopic clumps called plaques. The brain cells of persons with Alzheimer's disease also contain neurofribrillary tangles composed of a protein called *tau*. It is thought that beta amyloid and tau cause loss of synapse, the connections between brain cells.

Several forms of Alzheimer's disease are genetically transmitted or inherited. These inherited forms are usually associated with early onset Alzheimer's that occurs before the age of 50 and as early as 30. Less than 10% of all cases of Alzheimer's disease are inherited. All of the mutations to the DNA in the inherited forms involve the metabolism of beta-amyloid in some way. So even in the genetic forms, beta-amyloid remains central to the development of the disease. You can get more information about these mechanisms from your doctor or check with the organizations listed in this book.

How synapse loss affects brain function

As result of synapse and brain cell loss in certain parts of the brain, there is loss of the neurotransmitter acetylcholine, which transmits information along the nerves or neurons. This depletion contributes significantly to loss of memory and loss of capacity for attentiveness. Also, other brain chemicals, or neurotransmitters such as serotonin, GABA, somatostatin, and norepinephrine, are reduced by 50% or more. Elevated levels of the enzyme acetylcholinesterase in Alzheimer's disease breakdown acetylcholine and interfere with how the brain signals are sent between each other along the neurons.

Medical treatments for Alzheimer's disease may be prescribed by your physician. Currently there are two classes of medications approved by the Food and Drug Administration for treatment. These drugs are known as the acetyl cholinesterase inhibitors and glutamate inhibitors. They may be used singly or in combination. They are both modestly effective throughout the whole range of the disease, but are generally not prescribed for persons who have lost all ability to communicate or to care for themselves.

Your physician can prescribe medications based on your unique medical background. Like all medications, they must be monitored by a physician and may have side effects. See the appendix for a current list of prescription medications for treatment.

In the Alzheimer brain:

- The cortex shrinks, reflecting damage to areas involved in thinking, planning and remembering.

- Shrinkage is especially severe in the hippocampus, an area of the cortex that plays a key role in formation of new memories.

- Ventricles (fluid-filled spaces within the brain) grow larger.

The following is an image of brain tissue in a comparative cross section. This image illustrates the profound changes to the white and gray matter of the brain with Alzheimer's disease.

(The dark gray areas represent the gray matter and the lighter areas white matter)

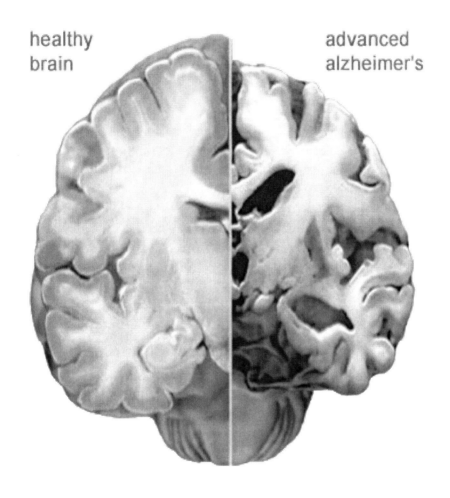

healthy
brain

advanced
alzheimer's

8
I hope they know....how to ask for help.

HOW MANY PEOPLE SUFFER in silence because of the fear they have about the unknown, or change, or anything that disturbs the status quo? Unconsciously, we understand that once change has been recognized then responsible action should follow. Denial may slow down a timely diagnosis and prevent early treatment.

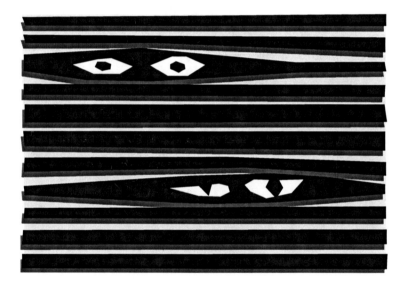

Denial is a great ally when fear has become a companion. Loved ones often hide the symptoms of Alzheimer's disease from others and even from their doctors, who may not be aware of subtle changes in behavior or personality or memory loss unless brought to their attention. The timely diagnosis is essential to plan ahead and begin early medical treatments; both can have a remarkable effect and make a substantial difference. Also finding support groups early on so they can be engaged from the beginning makes sense. This is the focus of early diagnosis and intervention and it gives the best chances for maintaining the best quality of life.

9

I hope they know....how important good nutrition will be.

WE ALL HAVE CONCERNS for getting the proper amount of vitamins and nutrients from our food. We try avoiding too much salt, fat, cholesterol and refined sugars and now along with fears about environmental pollutants and contaminants in our food, we seem to worry more than ever about what we eat. A healthy and balanced diet should be part of everyone's life style, but for the Alzheimer's patient, as the disease progresses, add new concerns about the appetite and eating patterns. They will change. Eventually even swallowing becomes difficult and food preparation will have to change when this happens. Foods will need to be bite size and have a texture to help with swallowing and avoid choking.

Getting enough daily liquids and water to prevent dehydration, which can worsen symptoms and exacerbate other medical problems, has no simple remedy. People with dementing illnesses may forget to eat and drink so they need to be prompted and offered food and water at customary times. Also if they are not eating well or irregularly you can try keeping a food diary. Weights should be taken so you can track if there is a significant reduction. Any weight loss greater than 10% of the existing body weight over 6 months is considered abnormal.

Some nutritional supplements are thought to slow down the disease but there are no current research studies to support this belief. Some supplements are listed in this book.

When to recognize swallowing difficulties and nutritional deficiencies is also covered. Caregivers should explore strategies for good nutrition with the doctor and medical support personnel.

10
I hope they know....agitation can come on suddenly.

MANY PEOPLE WITH DEMENTIA experience emotional distress or behavioral changes best summed up by the term *agitation.* Very mild agitation may seem like a personality change in which a person acts in ways that are uncharacteristic or inappropriate for him or her, such as being very stubborn, worried, or nervous. This may be related to some frustrating event, but more often seems to come out of the blue. More severe agitation forces caregivers to constantly supervise and reassure the person.

Agitation can be disruptive or even dangerous if it occurs while driving or in moments of vulnerability like crossing a busy street. Agitation tends to persist and to grow worse over time, and severe agitation is often the reason that families eventually decide to place loved ones in nursing homes.

Sundowning

Sundowning is a mild form of delirium that occurs in brain-damaged persons. We do not understand all of the mechanisms of sundowning but here are some examples of what it is and why it may happen. It consists of increasing confusion and agitation in the afternoons especially at dusk, in darkened rooms or unfamiliar places like a hospital or other care facility. Many persons with Alzheimer's disease become anxious. They think it is time to go home, feed the children, walk the dog, or close up at the office. Some trigger will "push the button in their brain" and it is impossible to redirect them away from their preoccupied thought. Sundowning is one of many mid- and late-stage symptoms. It may be brought on by fatigue, but can occur upon awakening after a nap. When sundowning occurs in a care facility, it may be related to the flurry of activity during staff shift changes. Staff arriving and leaving may cue some people with Alzheimer's to want to go home or to check on their children, or their pets—or they recall other behaviors that were appropriate in the late afternoon in their past. For many it was a time of action and transition but they do not remember or realize they no longer need to do anything.

Sundowning can occur anytime in the late day and early evening when there are increased shadows and low lighting. Soft music, beloved by the patient can be helpful and may restore calm. It is counter productive to insist on redirecting them to the "reality" of the situation. Also gentle touch can be used as well. These and many other non-medication strategies can be helpful, and should be explored for mild agitation and distress. They are discussed elsewhere in this book.

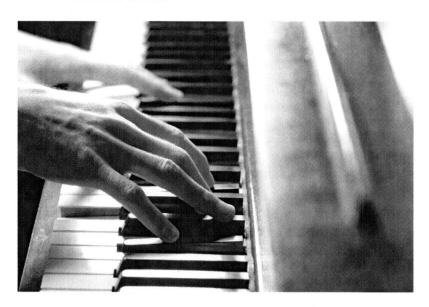

11

I hope they know....a person with early dementia can still drive.

THE DIAGNOSIS OF AN illness that leads to dementia is not in itself necessarily a reason to stop driving. A person diagnosed with such an illness may be able to continue driving for some time, although they must fulfill the state legal requirements to maintain their driving license. They need to have corrected vision and be medically fit to drive.

From a legal and a practical point of view, the question needs to be whether or not an individual is still able to drive safely. Your doctor can request that a driving test be performed to insure everyone's safety, but it is not the responsibility of the doctor alone. Learn about your state's driving regulations. In some states, California as an example, the physician must report a diagnosis of Alzheimer's to the health department, which then reports it to the department of motor vehicles. That agency then may revoke the person's license. Your local Alzheimer's Association may have information available on driving regulations in your state. Your doctor can get the information for you as well.

The appendix has a worksheet that can help you decide if it is time for an Alzheimer's patient to stop driving. These items listed are only warning signs and high risk signs for the elderly in general. They should be evaluated with real concern but recognizing and balancing independence issues with public safety concerns. When any person's condition deteriorates to the point where they are unsafe on the roads, regardless of their age or medical condition, they must stop driving and family must support this decision. For many people diagnosed with illness that lead to dementia, this is very difficult to accept because it diminishes freedom and often is the first step that makes them codependent on others.

Remember, even for experienced drivers, driving is a complicated task that requires a split-second combination of complex thought processes and manual skills. To drive, a person needs to be able to make sense of and respond to everything they see and hear in daylight and in the darkness. Today, in most states it is legal for cell phones to be used while people drive and talk at the same time holding the cell phone in their hand. Other states have or will soon have the hands free law for cell phone use. Cell phone use can make defensive driving even more of a challenge as drivers have divided attention. The traffic laws are by state and you cannot follow them if you do not know them. Ask at you local department of vehicle registration or the National Highway Traffic and Safety Administration.

Simply to 'read the road', to follow road signs, to anticipate and react quickly to the actions of other road users and to take appropriate action to avoid accidents, is not as easy as it once was. To remember where one is going and how to return is also necessary. As dementia progresses it has serious effects on memory, perception and the ability to perform even simple tasks. People with illnesses that cause dementia will, therefore, eventually lose the ability to drive. The stage at which this happens will be different for each person.

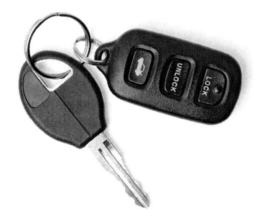

Resources and Further Reading

Driving pools may be a resource in your community. If you want to learn more about driving pools, check with your local Retirement Association. Church groups also often provide transportation services. The Association for Driver Rehabilitation Specialists has some interesting fact sheets relating to medical conditions and driving. The Association is a good resource for information on driving and aging as is the National Association of Area Agencies on Aging. You can also find services by state to help you with carpooling and drive sharing.

Taking away the keys is to insure everyone's safety and is the responsibility of the family.

Contact The National Center on Senior Transportation. http://seniortransportation.easterseals. com

12

I hope they know....is the person unsure of their ability to drive?

FREQUENT MINOR ACCIDENTS, OR getting lost often, or simply running out of gas more than once might all be good signals that is time to stop driving. Look for signs of unsafe driving such as forgetting how to locate familiar places, failing to observe traffic signs, making slow or poor decisions in traffic, driving at an inappropriate speed, or becoming angry or confused while driving. Keep a written record of your observations to share with the person affected with early dementia or Alzheimer's disease, and other family members and health care professionals. Have the person's driving ability tested. Some state agencies have special drive tests to determine how well a person sees, judges distance and responds to traffic.

The National Highway Traffic and Safety Administration has self tests and physical tests and information to help you. Ask the person who administers the test to explain the results to you and to the person with dementia. If your state does not offer special testing, alternative assessments (generally fee-for-service) may be available. Your local Alzheimer's Association may be able to provide a list of these. "At the Crossroads: A Guide to Alzheimer's disease, Dementia, and Driving," is a publication that provides strategies and greater information.

For most of us, driving is something we take for granted and is part of our collective, social identification. Giving it up, is one of the most difficult aspects in the middle stages of the disease as the loss of driving cuts back independence. It is best to get ongoing support from the family and health care professionals if resistance to leaving the keys and car is a problem.

Many urban communities have shuttle services for the elderly. These driving resources are unique to each community and can be discovered with the help of your doctor or elder service planner and your local Alzheimer's Association Chapter.

13

I hope they know....how upset and upsetting people can be.

ONCE THE DIAGNOSIS OF Alzheimer's disease is made and other persons important to the patient are made aware, most will act with compassion, but some may react in ways that are not useful. They may feel fear of the unknown (or what they imagine will happen), or may see the affected person as the victim of an over anxious family member. They may become angry and blame other family members for exaggerating the problem.

Unfortunately, not everyone handles frightening things well. The changes and responsibilities that any significant illness creates for families will challenge their time and needs, which must be met and balanced with other parts of their lives. This can often cause family strain. Your relationship to the person with Alzheimer's disease and other family members will change, whether you are a brother, daughter, nephew, friend or spouse. Although you cannot control how other people react, you can promote education and information sharing. If others in the family do not react supportively, you may feel alone with the disease or within your family.

Educating your self and family about the disease and the care options makes sense and will reduce family conflict and stress for the person who becomes the primary caregiver. Developing a good support group is necessary, whether through the Alzheimer's association, church, or family.

The love that others feel is often hard to show in the face of fear of the disease.

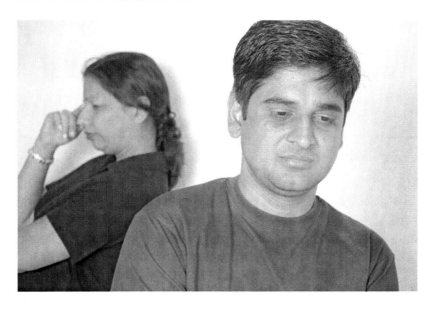

14
What Is Quality of Life and Where Can It Be Found?
By Myron Weiner, M.D.

MUCH HAS BEEN WRITTEN about quality of life, but we lack a good definition for this often-used term. Possible substitute words are happiness or serenity. A popular song from a few years ago (maybe many years ago) had lyrics including the phrase "Happiness is...(long pause) ...different things to different people; that's what happiness is!" But as each of us has learned from experience, happiness is more often pursued than found. How about serenity? I can actually define serenity. It is the ability or the quality of being undisturbed by the daily ups and downs of life. My own view is that a person's quality of life is measured by his comfort with who he is, what he does, and how he feels both physically and emotionally. Even while people become unable to do or to remember names or events, they still can feel physical or emotional discomfort, and can still feel comfortable and comforted, and they are often serene.

What is the effect of Alzheimer's disease on quality of life?

How can there be quality of life for persons with Alzheimer's disease? Alzheimer's disease has been described in the medical literature as a fatal disease, but in my experience over the past 22 years of observing and working with persons having the disease, Alzheimer's is a chronic illness much like diabetes or high blood pressure. Patients and their families learn to live with it. It is hard for many of us to understand how it could be possible to have a high quality of life while experiencing the losses brought about by Alzheimer's disease; progressive loss of memory and other mental functions; knowing less than we used to, being able to learn less, and being less able to assert our preferences (or objections), and having less of our own way? How does a person live comfortably without doing the sort of work or hobbies that formerly made up a personal identity? We are all familiar with the notion that a person is what he does. What happens to our comfort with ourselves when we can no longer do the activities that formerly defined us, such being a mother or grandmother? How do people like mothers and grandmothers who see themselves as caregivers make the transition to what we clumsily call a care recipient and what we might better simply call a loved one?

As everything else in life, having Alzheimer's disease is both a threat and an opportunity. It gives families and patients the opportunity to deal with life in a way that might have otherwise been overlooked. Because having Alzheimer's disease pushes us more and more to live in the present, families and patient can ask themselves what do I value that I can have or do today? While patients cannot learn new sets of skills, they can live each day fully, using the aspects of themselves that do not depend on job skills or earning income.

With Alzheimer's disease can come increased quality of life. If mother forgets or is unaware of the health problems of son John and daughter-in-law Mary, she has less cause to worry. With relinquishment of the checkbook to another family member, she can release her concern over finances and have a sense that they are in good hands. It may be hard to believe, but quality of life is partly related to our ability to ignore, overlook, or minimize troubling issues such as physical health or the ability to perform complex tasks. By contrast, adults who are prone to depression frequently have a more realistic view of the world and their own life situation than those who are not subject to depression. We actually need our rosy colored glasses to make life tolerable.

The threat of Alzheimer's disease is losing contact with ourselves and others; the opportunity is to strengthen that bond and to develop a new, ever-changing identity that conforms with who we are and not whom we wish or feel we ought to be. Alzheimer's disease is simply another life experience to which one accommodates and by which one is shaped. But a good cup of coffee is still a good cup of coffee regardless of a person's ability to manage financial affairs. The warmth of the sun on a cool day still has the same quality whether or not we recognize the warmth as coming from the sun. Our ability to appreciate a smile and a warm greeting persists beyond the point that we can recognize who is smiling and greeting us. The appreciation of tender touch is unchanged, and the ability to love and to receive love remains.

Quality of life for persons with Alzheimer's disease has much less to do with what they are able to accomplish than it does a sense of being untroubled and living in a predictable environment. Sameness becomes security, not monotony. Simplicity in daily living gives a sense of comfort rather than loss.

How can we help maintain quality of life of persons with Alzheimer's disease?

We can offer our loved ones affection and sameness in a physical and emotional setting that matches their needs. For example, many families notice that their affected loved one becomes very uncomfortable at large family gatherings, but is quite comfortable with one-on-one visitation. So, if large holiday gatherings are an important family tradition, the person with Alzheimer's disease can be allowed to watch television in a quite room and be visited by family members one at a time, sparing the confusion of many persons speaking at once. We can avoid correcting loved ones when they misname someone or recall a fact incorrectly. We can fill in for their inabilities instead of pushing them harder to perform at the level they did before. On the other hand, we can respect the decision making capacity they still maintain. We can offer the unconditional love that many of us experienced from our parents when we were young children and that we all still need to a certain extent. We can recognize that our loved ones' future is our present, and that this is where we need to live, whether through exchange of words, glances or touch. Quality of life can be found anywhere, including special care units in nursing homes and in hospice care, regardless of setting. It is the coming together of people on common ground with mutual respect, each offering what he or she can offer.

15
I hope they know....how important grooming will become.

THERE WILL BE A slow change in the appearance of the patient with Alzheimer's disease. It is important that they follow their routine and get up everyday, brush their hair, shave, wash their face, and change into clean, fresh smelling clothing. It is important that dental health and hygiene are maintained. Some days there will be incontinence and gradually clothes will have to be changed more frequently. Special toileting and precautions will begin. That usually happens in the late stages, but if incontinence is already a problem, it will get worse. Soiling is one of the biggest stressors for family and caregivers. A person who has soiled may feel their dignity is challenged. They may feel stress over the encroaching reality of dependency that will require a loved one to clean and change them. Many do not accept this situation, and daily home health aides may be required at this point, or some other solution and strategy explored.

It will be helpful in the beginning that *your* someone with Alzheimer's disease look their best, it will buoy your spirits and theirs and keep the routine going for them. It is a time for photographs and a time to remember who you are and what you and your companion or family look and feel like now.

We are all beautiful!

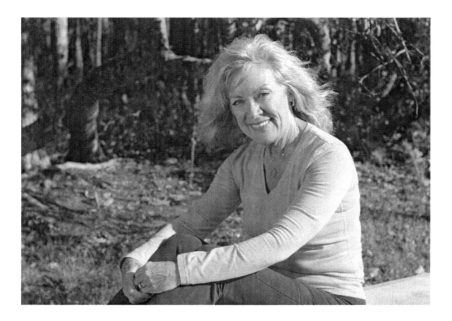

16
I hope they know....how important the routine will become.

MOST OF US LIKE our things put in the same place. Most of us like to eat at the same time, watch the same programs or go to bed and fall asleep with a good book. For the Alzheimer's patient routine becomes more important. Creating calm surroundings and keeping a routine can have an enormously positive impact. As the disease progresses, frustration at misplacing things can generate agitation, fear, suspiciousness and anxiety. The disease symptoms and the subsequent suspicion and paranoia can become very hard on caretakers, family and friends. This happens more frequently as short-term memory begins to fail. Keep a routine, keep rooms well lit and minimize noise to create a calm surrounding.

Don't try to change too many things at the same time. Assistive technology is just that, a tool that can assist in managing many of the early symptoms. Try to add these devices and technologies gradually so they may become part of the daily routine. Helpful assistive technologies are covered in this book.

17
Did He Forget Again?

NOW I MOSTLY FORGET
where I left my keys.
But why should I drive,
if they said I can't see?

I didn't forget I was married,
then I divorced.
Right after the war,
time followed its course
and healed my wounds.

They say I forget
the usual things,
how to comb my hair
or put on a tie,
make my bed
or get the mail.
Then they shout
stay out of the way!
But who cares of these things?
They belong
to yesterday.

Zoë Lewis M.D., © 2007

18

I hope they know....how visiting with friends and family can help.

MANY CAREGIVERS WILL BEGIN to feel isolated, not able to leave the home for fear of something happening. Just having company and someone to laugh with, cry with and share a meal with can make a smile or bring a laugh or a tear that needs to come. It may be hard to ask for company, some of us are not blessed with family nearby or friends that can visit as often as we like. Get involved with the organizations that can help you with volunteers. Look into the local day programs, or find out about respite care if your loved one needs supervision 24/7. Don't wait until you are burned out, frustrated and angry. Learn how to be candid and let people know when you need them. If you are in an urban area, there are many resources. Rural areas present more of a challenge, yet programs and outreach groups exist everywhere. You may find help through the Veterans Administration, or seniors groups at the local hospital or your religious center. Ask your doctor for help in finding support if you are isolated. Join groups and continue with your fun activities, it will keep your mental health balanced.

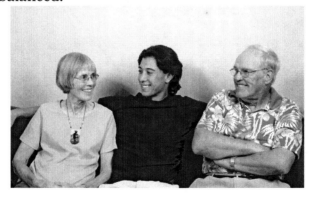

19
I hope they know....the end may be years away.

SOME OF THE FIRST QUESTIONS upon diagnosis are "How long will I live? How does the disease progress? What stage am I?"

Alzheimer's disease is a slow disease, starting with mild memory problems and ending with severe brain damage. On average, Alzheimer's disease patients live from 8 to 10 years after they are diagnosed, though affected persons can survive as many as 20 years. People with dementia lose their abilities at different rates. These prognosis and staging questions are best answered considering certain facts. For example, whether there is another illness that is coexisting that can hasten a decline. Medical professionals track the progression of Alzheimer's disease by stages. The progression can be described as a series of stages providing a guide to the pattern of the disease, which can help when making care decisions. There are two staging systems. One staging system explains the disease in three stages: early, middle and late. Another staging system, often used by medical professionals, is the Global Deterioration Scale (also called the Reisberg Scale or GDS). This scale divides the disease into seven stages. The Global Deterioration Scale and the Three Stage System are listed in the Appendix.

Staging systems are also one of the many determinants used by medical doctors to declare eligibility for hospice services if they are desired or suggested then elected by the patient and family. Whichever staging system is used it's important to remember that the disease affects each person differently. The length of each stage, including other variables of symptom presentation, are unique for each person.

No one clear event marks when one stage ends and another begins. In many cases, stages will overlap. Some people experience many of the symptoms in each stage, while others experience only a few. There may be fluctuations from week to week with a person appearing more confused one day, for example, and less so another. Other times the symptoms may plateau for quite some time with no further decline. This is another challenge for caretakers, but over time, the stage becomes apparent. It is important to remember that the approach to care as the disease progresses is to enhance the individual's quality of life and manage new symptoms as they arise.

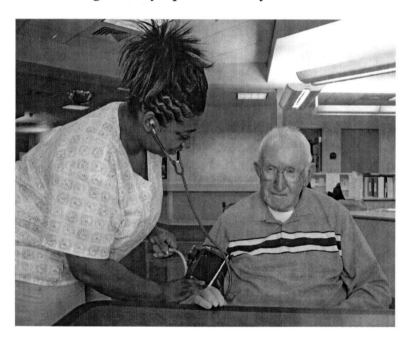

20
I hope they know....sexual intimacy and relationships will change.

WE ALL NEED LOVE and we need to feel loved. Everyone has a need for companionship and physical intimacy. People with Alzheimer's disease or a related dementia are no different. There is little research about Alzheimer's disease and dementia illness and the expression of sexuality, sexual desire and the need for intimacy, yet we all know this is an important aspect of an adult life.

So what happens?

Sexuality does change when someone has Alzheimer's disease. It changes with any disease. It changes as we age. The relationship changes as well, as do your roles within the relationship to meet the demands of the disease. The diminishing ability of the impaired partner takes the healthy partner into new areas of need and service. The physical, psychological and social changes in turn mean either partner can find responding to sexual advances difficult. It is a perfectly normal reaction. This is perhaps because the sexual side of a relationship is often one of the first things that are changed by any illness. There are numerous reasons for this. The effects of the disease, possible medication side effects, and the effects from other disease processes can impact on how you view one another sexually.

Sexuality and Disease

Because Alzheimer's disease affects people in different ways, how an individual behaves, just as people's personalities are different, remains individual. Some people have increased and some decreased interest in sex. It can be the reverse behavior from when they were well. Often the resulting sexual behavior can be quite different than from pre-Alzheimer's diagnosis. The progression of the disease and its effect on the brain means that although sexual desire may be felt, the response may create difficulties in expressing affect. Libido may also be affected by medications. The loss of self esteem is another one of the changes that can influence sexual behavior.

In contrast, decreased inhibitions, inappropriate behavior and reduced sensitivity to the partner all mean potential difficulties as the disease progresses.

Talk about your feelings with your partner. Allow them to share their feelings. If there is new impotence, reassure them. Show affection and love through touch, kisses and words. If sexual advances and behavior are creating problems for your relationship or aggression is beginning to take place, then you must get help.

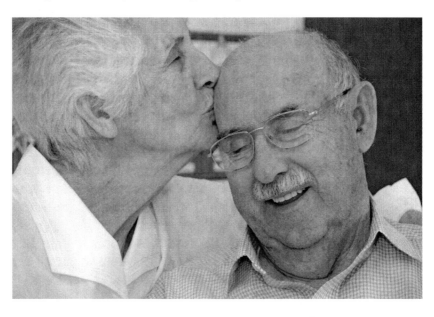

There is a section in part two for suggestions on inappropriate behaviors. Your doctor or health care team will be able to help out as well. This is not something to be ashamed of, but discussed openly with your doctor so they can help.

21
I hope they know....the link between loneliness and Alzheimer's disease.

WE ALL NEED FRIENDS and healthy interactions with others to maintain our emotional health and wellbeing. Research on loneliness and Alzheimer's disease now suggests that people who are persistently lonely may be more vulnerable to the age related effects of dementia illnesses. Studies have shown that social isolation, or having few interactions with others, is associated with an increased risk of dementia and cognitive decline. However, little is known about emotional isolation. This refers to feeling alone rather than being alone.

Keeping active physically and intellectually during the retirement years is not a new message. Making new friends and avoiding complete social isolation may actually prevent or slow down dementia illnesses. Alzheimer's day programs maintain social interactions and can provide the activities that can stimulate, challenge and even give joy to those whose interactions were limited in an isolated home environment. New friendships can be made.

A friend is one of life's great gifts.

Also new evidence suggests physical exercise and activity is as important as mental and social activity in preventing and slowing the progression of Alzheimer's disease.

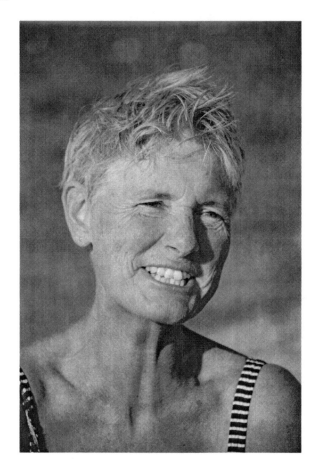

22

I hope they know....medical research is ongoing.

DEVELOPING PREVENTATIVE OR CURATIVE measures is the task at hand for the medical community. The earliest diagnosis and treatment, together with developing an awareness of new medications and new therapies may have the greatest impact on maintaining a good quality of life for the longest period.

Worldwide, networking in both private sector and non profit funding programs promote the intense research effort to understand the mechanisms of the disease and find possible cures. Nearly every major pharmaceutical company is working on this problem, as are private organizations, as well as the federal government. Promising treatments need to be tested and, if safe and effective, made available to the public as rapidly as possible.

Without research studies to quantify and qualify an intervention, observations are anecdotal. For example, no published study directly compares the current medications for Alzheimer's treatment. Because they work in a similar way, it is not expected that switching from one of these drugs to another will produce significantly different results. However, a patient may respond better to one drug than another. The impact of nonmedical treatments on quality of life is another area in need of greater research efforts.

23
I hope they know....alternative dietary supplements and treatments exist.

THERE ARE MANY CHOICES of both drugs and nutritional supplements available for patients with Alzheimer's disease. Nutritional supplements are thought by many persons to have benefits, but have not undergone scientific studies to suport their use. An aggressive program of dietary supplementation should not be started without the supervision of a qualified physician. Several of the nutrients suggested may have adverse effects. These are some of the most commonly suggested today.

- Curcumin—900 to 1800 milligrams (mg) daily
- EPA/DHA—1400 mg daily of EPA and 1000 mg daily of DHA
- Vitamin E—400 international units (IU) daily (with 200 mg of gamma-tocopherol)
- Vitamin C—1 to 3 grams daily
- Ginkgo biloba—120 mg daily
- Acetyl-L-carnitine arginate—750 to 2000 mg daily
- CoQ10—100 to 600 mg daily
- N-acetylcysteine—600 mg daily
- Aged garlic—1200 mg daily
- Vinpocetine—15 to 20 mg daily
- Green tea extract (93 percent polyphenols)—725 mg daily
- B vitamins—A full complement of B vitamins (including folate, vitamin B6, and vitamin B12) to lower homocysteine. Specific suggested doses include 1000 micrograms (mcg) of vitamin B12, 250 mg of vitamin B6, and 800 mcg of folic acid.

- **Niacin**—Up to 800 mg daily. Start slowly and take with food to avoid flushing.
- **Melatonin**—1 to 3 mg each night
- **DHEA**—15 to 75 mg daily. Have blood tested in 3 to 6 weeks to determine optimal dose.
- **Huperzine**—50 mcg up to four times per week
- **Blueberry extract**—500 to 2000 mg daily. If you eat blueberries, you don't need to take this much blueberry extract.
- **Grape seed extract**—100 mg daily

Nutrients such as phosphatidylserine-DHA (PS-DHA), glycerophosphorylcholine (GPC), phosphatidylserine, vinpocetine, and ashwagandha, are available in multi-nutrient mixes.

Please check with your doctor first before you take anything. Many other supplements exist and this is not an exhaustive list.

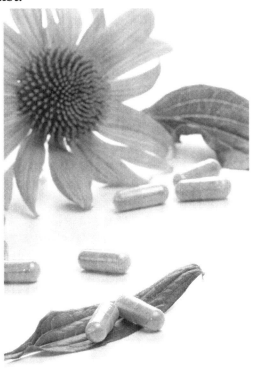

24
I hope they know....art therapy improves the quality of life.

ART THERAPY BECAME ESTABLISHED as a mental health profession in the 1930s. It is now practiced in hospitals, clinics, public and community agencies, wellness centers, educational institutions, homeless shelters, businesses and private practices. Art therapy has found a role among a wide range of individuals suffering with many emotional and physical ailments. It involves the application of a variety of art modalities including drawing, painting, clay and sculpture and other arts and crafts techniques.

Certain individuals with dementia have displayed a new interest and ability in art in the beginning stages of the disease through the end stages. Day programs using art and creative therapies for people with Alzheimer's may also help to eliminate the stigma often associated with the disease. Art therapy enables the expression of inner thoughts or feelings when verbalization is difficult or not possible. Especially for the late stage nonverbal Alzheimer or dementia patient, it can improve the quality of life and reconnect a dementia patient with the outside world. The aesthetic aspect of the creation of art is thought to lift one's mood, boost self-awareness and improve self-esteem. Art therapy also allows the opportunity to exercise the eyes and hands, improve eye-hand coordination and stimulate neurological pathways from the brain to the hands. Art therapy may aid in stress reduction and relaxation for the care giver as well.

No one knows exactly how art taps into physical and intellectual memories muddled by neurodegenerative diseases. But scientists suspect that the process allows people to find alternate routes to misplaced memories.

Information in the brain appears to be organized much like the entries in the old-fashioned library card catalog. A book will have one card as its main entry, but also several others organized by category linking back to the book. Similarly, a memory of an event can be reached directly but also through its links with other information stored in the brain. Remembering often takes this route, linking similar objects in a category. Recall for example when you forgot a name but recognized it began with a certain letter, like B. For this reason as you start drawing a picture of your family vacation spot, whether it is a beach, farm or mountainside ski area, suddenly you might have access to memories of events that occurred there. It's not surprising that drawing, or painting works to bring back memories. The process of creating images from one's own unconscious is even more powerful than looking at the painting of another. Both can evoke responses, but the process of creating the image is more likely to evoke personal memories and bring a sense of improved mood. The end result, the drawing, painting, or clay sculpture is what matters. Also the substance of the image can tell us a lot about what is going on for the "artist" emotionally.

The Museum of Modern Art recently began to experiment with short, focused tours, working with an Alzheimer's care company called Hearthstone, based in Lexington, Mass. *Meet Me at MoMA*, is a pioneering program for individuals with Alzheimer's and other forms of dementia and their family members and care partners at The Museum of Modern Art in New York.

The Boston Museum of Fine Arts began to reach out to Alzheimer's patients more than five years ago, offering tours alongside those for other disabled groups. The Bruce Museum of Arts and Science in Greenwich, Conn., also offers tours, in addition to conducting a program in which it sends educators to Alzheimer's care facilities to help with art therapy.

Perhaps in your area there are museum programs for people with Alzheimer's disease. Museum educators can view these programs as potentially satisfying experiences for people without full access to their memory and can give those living with the degenerative disease an expressive outlet and forum for dialogue with caregivers. It also gives the Alzheimer's patient the opportunity to be visually stimulated in the setting of museum galleries.

25
Art Therapy for Quality of Life
By Elizabeth Cockey, MAT

ACCORDING TO THE AMERICAN Art Therapy Association, art therapy first emerged as a profession in the 1930s and has been increasingly used by healthcare professionals to improve the physical, mental and emotional well-being of children and adults in a variety of settings. Along with this, a growing number of long-term care facilities and adult day programs are tapping this creative process for individuals with Alzheimer's disease and other dementias.

Whether done in a community setting or at home, art therapy provides an enriched environment that can excite the imagination, even in the most severely impaired individual. Creating art stimulates regions in the brain that affect memory and coordination that have become inactive due to cognitive impairment disorders. When Alzheimer's disease strips individuals of verbal skills, this recreational activity provides an alternative means by which they can express themselves in a non-threatening and comfortable way. And it can also help someone recover the use of motor skills in the same manner as physical rehabilitation.

Although the impact of art therapy is still being studied, a handful of researchers have found positive and measurable results when it is utilized for individuals with dementia. Moreover, art therapists informally report the effectiveness of art making. It is possible to stimulate creativity through the implementation of simple games and exercises that are designed to be "failure free" art-making processes with people who have dementia. While the arts and creative expression are open to everyone, arts programs work best if staff, family or volunteers have some training.

One of the big challenges in encouraging the use of arts in dementia care is to convince the staff at long term care facilities that people with all levels of dementia can be creative.

Personal Experiences

I have witnessed dramatic changes in individuals who participated in art therapy, many that had previously remained secluded within the confines of their long-term care facility rooms. Some clients literally crawl out of their shells, while others who are unable to communicate through words, express delight, appear more relaxed or exhibit less behavioral problems. Some even become boastful: when his peers recognized his paintings, one individual with dementia proclaimed, "Wait till you see my etchings!"

One such individual, I'll call Eleanor preferred to sit alone in her room after she was moved into the dementia care unit at an assisted living facility. She ignored activities, rarely had visitors and gradually stopped communicating entirely. By the time she was introduced to my art therapy program it was thought that she was completely deaf; she barely responded when spoken to and was despondent. Then the residence added my "experimental" art therapy program to the weekly calendar of events. Would Eleanor and some other women who spent much of their time pacing or watching television get into the creative spirit?

I began by drawing outlines of fruit, vegetables, flowers and other objects they would recognize with black paint and guided the residents to color them in with non-toxic tempera paint—almost like paint-by-number. At first Eleanor would have none of it. She looked up and shook her head back and forth, then stood up to leave. Two other women followed. Together with an activity assistant, we gently led them back to start again. It took a bit of coaxing but we managed to place paintbrushes in their hands and showed them how to move their brushes across the paper.

Staying within the outlines that had already been drawn in, they were able to fill in each piece of fruit, or a flower within a very short time. The women started to smile. More sessions followed, and the resulting paintings were framed and hung up in the hallways for everyone to admire.

With each passing week, Eleanor no longer had to be coaxed out of her room for the one-hour art therapy, and her paintings and other projects became a source of conversation among the residents in that unit. Eleanor began to talk again, even telling many delightful stories about her childhood. One day during our art session I asked Eleanor why she hadn't spoken before. Eleanor thought a moment and then started to laugh. "I just never had anything to say," she answered. Thanks to art therapy, her life and the lives of the other residents had started to change.

Together in a group setting, participants often develop a newfound sense of camaraderie. They get to know more about one another, translating into better relationships and friendships. Teamwork and conversation encourage compliments, which boost self-esteem. What I have discovered in working with individuals with slight to mid-range dementia is that art therapy combined with psychotherapy and medication resulted in improved cognitive memory function; especially with short-term memory. I also noticed that the residents I worked with had better hand-to-eye coordination with small motor skills applications. Many became less dependent upon medication for depression and other stress-related disorders; including a reduction in delusional thinking, especially in the afternoon when some are subject to behavioral disturbances, commonly known as sun downing.

Even with people affected by Alzheimer's I find that what remains intact is the ability to appreciate beauty, to know what's good and what's not so good, especially in the visual. That coupled with the ability to create beautiful things has a therapeutic effect. Individuals who have lost nearly everything: their independence, memories, the ability to express themselves fully, or to have a coherent conversation can feel productive again. The truth is that art brings out the best in everybody at all ages and stages of development. Art can become the connection that unites those who can't walk, who are incontinent, confused, non-verbal or can't hear what you're saying.

Communication Benefits

It is possible and sometimes desirable to relay information non-verbally. To better illustrate this point, I will tell you about a group of Russian-speaking women with Alzheimer's disease that I work with. First of all, none of them speak English; and I don't speak Russian. I was first introduced to the group because they needed something to do and the facility was at a loss about how to create an activity for them that would be engaging and enjoyable that they could comprehend without it becoming necessary to understand English. I began by placing a blank piece of paper in front of each of them and then handed each one a picture of scenery, or a building. Next I painted a rough sketch of the picture and outlined a portion in the color I wanted them to paint with; using green for the lawn, blue for the sky, red for the barn, and so forth. It didn't take long before they were filling in between the lines, or taking initiative, anxious for the next color. They were grinning and singing; trying to teach me Russian words, holding onto my hand.

For some individuals, just like the Russian women, familiar images can spark an emotional connection and release a memory that generates positive feelings. Others get that reassurance by staring at pictures with large areas of color; or religious iconography. Which art is the right prescription for health and healing is, as one might expect in the eye of the beholder. Landscapes seem to work well for many individuals, perhaps because at some point in life we likely had the opportunity to enjoy nature or the outdoors. Where rational language and factual memory have failed people with dementia, the arts offer an avenue for communication and connection with caregivers, loved ones and the greater world.

The Science Behind Art Therapy

Art-making or the act of creating involves every single part of the brain. It stimulates our neurogenic pathways while it stimulates our neurohormonal production and that makes us feel good. During a period of creativity, a network in the lateral frontal cortex of one or both hemispheres of the brain is stimulated. In a study completed by Singer in 2002, *"What makes a creative genius tick?"* It was found that creativity is not only thinking outside the box but also feeling emotions outside the box. The neurochemistry associated with this level of thought stimulates an emotional reaction. Creative thinking also encourages the formation of new neurons and this can be considered positive feedback for a dementing illnesses. The artist hones his or her talent by repeated practice, and the ability to be stimulated by the creative process eventually becomes ingrained within the artist's neural pathways. The new circuitry helps to increase the potential to feel inspired and to transcend physical and psychological pain through engagement in creative work.

When individuals engage in art-making, whether it be painting, sculpting or construction, they realize that there is more to life than just their own circumstances. My experience in working with Alzheimer's and dementia patients is backed up by a report released last year by the National Endowment for the Arts on the impact of arts programs on older Americans. The study found that seniors who participate in weekly arts programs reported better health, fewer doctor visits, and less medication usage than those who don't. In order for arts programs to successfully compete for time and money, we need research that clearly demonstrates the benefits of arts programs to help provide a quality of life for people with dementia. The arts will not provide a cure, but the art programs I have facilitated demonstrate dramatic improvements in quality of life: easing depression, improving coordination and relieving boredom to name a few.

The Emotional Benefits of Art Therapy

There are so many things that the dying and the infirm don't have choices about, like daily living and activities associated with living such as dressing, going to the bathroom, eating, receiving medications and in some cases medical procedures. Instead of lying in bed with a sense of hopelessness or dread, art programs can give each individual something to look forward to and the ability to make choices, and instill a sense of purpose. The choices may be simple such as what color to use, but each individual can take an active role in creating something. Art programs can provide an opportunity to make choices in an environment where choices are otherwise limited.

For art therapists and activity staff is it important to realize that some elderly clients are often unable to fully execute their creative ideas, so they require the use of the therapist's mobility, imagination or technical knowledge. Edith Kramer (1986) illustrated how the art therapist's artistic abilities and imagination are used to empathically carry out the creative intention of the client. Naming this type of therapeutic assistance the "third hand", Kramer described it not as an intervention, but rather an extension of the client. In this manner, the art therapist must rely on his or her own artistic abilities to execute the artistic intentions of the client, yet must subdue his or her own artistic style when carrying out the work of the client. The loss of physical faculties, as a result of disease or disability, may significantly impair an individual's ability to engage in self-expression. Adapting an art technique for a physically impaired client gives that person the experience of tapping into the senses.

Successful art therapy with older adults should stem from the belief that aging provides the opportunity to discover life's meaning in the art-making process. Nurturing ideas through imagination and visualization and then putting them into practice through art, like painting or sculpting brings about a greater sense of self and accomplishment to each and every individual who participates. In Erik Erikson's model of the stages of the life cycle, the eighth and final stage of growth is described as the individual's bringing together his/her past, present and future. In Erikson's estimation, older people who successfully integrate the past, present and future are able to face their own mortality with wisdom instead of despair. In the creative older adult, this life stage is reflected in the convergence of self-knowledge and mastery of creative technique, as evidenced in the artwork of Renoir, Matisse, O'Keeffe and Monet.

For families, art offers a viable activity that can bring family members together via a new channel of expression especially when verbal communication fails. It might just be the interaction for younger children who are frightened by grandmas' illness. If your loved one is in a long-term care facility or nursing home, visiting during a time when an activity such as art therapy is underway can be beneficial on several fronts. Staff will usually welcome the additional pair of hands, and it gives you and your loved one something to do together.

Home Projects

At home you can plan an art activity to do together on a regular basis. You do not have to go very far to find the right materials either. Some like clay, paint and papier-mâché can be made in the kitchen; others such as scraps of material can be found around the house; and some basics like large white sheets of construction paper and inexpensive paintbrushes can be purchased at a local craft store, or a large supermarket. Other useful items to have on hand are: newspapers to cover tabletops; brown postal paper to paint on; old cloth napkins, buttons and ribbon to fashion into pillows; and Elmer's glue to attach pieces of material in lieu of stitching. Whether you choose drawing, sculpting or another type of art project, try to remember that it is the process, not the finished product. Emotional gratification and the ability to share something are the best effects of art therapy and what count most.

As a professional art therapist, caregiver, or family member we all have a wonderful opportunity to make a difference through the creative process. Your loved one may not be able to walk, hear what you are saying or understand the world around them, but through the creative process it is possible to reconnect and have a life that is worth living. I believe that doing art makes everyone better, one brushstroke at a time.

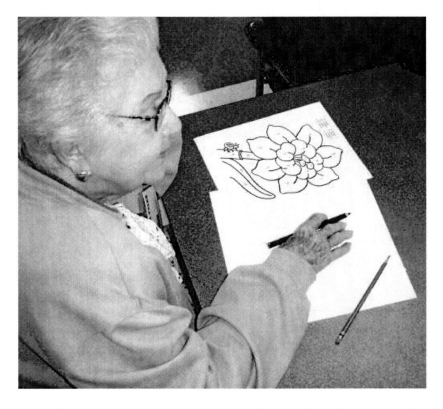

Artistic expression can be as simple as choosing one color over another. Zoë Lewis© 2007

26

I hope they know....what is an advance directive?

ADVANCE DIRECTIVES ARE LEGAL documents that allow you to plan and make known your healthcare wishes in the event that you are unable to communicate. Advance directives consist of a living will and a medical power of attorney. A living will describes your wishes regarding medical care. A medical power of attorney allows you to appoint a person to make health care decisions for you in case you are unable to speak for yourself.

When patients are diagnosed with Alzheimer's disease or a dementia illness, they will need to make aware their thoughts regarding the extent and duration of medical treatments they will receive as their illness progresses. This is a very difficult task in the initial period following an early stage diagnosis because it forces the individual and their family to confront the progressive aspects of the disease. These considerations need to occur long before the significant changes of Alzheimer's have occurred. However, timing in this instance is the issue; advance directives must be addressed while competency is not challenged.

The whether to continue medical treatment and if so, how much treatment, and for how long, is difficult at best. In these instances, patients rely on their physicians or other trusted health professionals for guidance. In the best of circumstances, the patient, the family, and the physician have held discussions about treatment options, including the length and invasiveness of treatment, chance of success, overall prognosis, and the patient's quality of life during and after the treatment. Ideally, these discussions would continue as the patient's condition changes, however with Alzheimer's disease the mental capability wanes over time, therefore making these personal choices and thoughtfulness about the situation imperative as soon as the diagnosis is made. The choice for life-sustaining medical care, including but not limited to the use of semi-permanent feeding tubes and mechanical ventilators or breathing machines are such issues. The addition of apparatus for many represents a turning point in "quality of life" considering once mechanical breathing or tube feeding is initiated, it is rarely, if ever, disconnected in advanced dementia patients.

Other issues are ongoing antibiotic therapy to fight recurrent infections from indwelling tubing like Foley catheters and IV lines, blood thinners requiring blood level monitoring or recurrent blood product transfusions. These are only a handful of the life support treatments that should all be considered by the patient when they are still able to make decisions and plan for the future.

A frank discussion about the implications of medical orders like DNR (do not resuscitate) or DNI (do not intubate) should also be held with your doctor. Frequently, however, such discussions are not held. If the patient becomes incapacitated due to his illness, the patient's family and physician must make decisions based on what they think the patient would want. This is the law, however many problems still can occur with differences of opinion between family members and the next of kin-healthcare surrogate as disease progresses and emotional factors begin to weight in. Consider the famous state and federal Supreme Court cases in the past 20 years. Now the right to life and right to die debates make international news with ardent stories of ongoing legal battles surrounding these issues. If no next of kin is alive or willing, then a court appointed health care surrogate is determined.

It is best to leave advance directives to guide professional care and guide loved ones in the oversight of the care regardless of the illness, but especially for Alzheimer's patients. Your doctor will have the printed materials and resources necessary and help you make these decisions. These are often difficult conversations and may require multiple visits. It is best to have open and even recorded conversations together within the family, especially if wishes and views about care provisions differ. Ethical concerns about competency can be avoided if these steps are taken as soon as the diagnosis is made, if in an early stage. Once mental capacity is challenged then competency can become a complicating factor, voiding a directive.

Keep in mind as well, that laws differ from state to state and there is no one "form". If you live in one state and have a vacation home in another, make sure you check with your doctor to fulfill the obligations for both states with your living will document. Legal advice is not necessary but there are elder law specialists that can provide additional services.

Whatever an individual decides, it should be respected and honored by loved ones and family. Advance directives can spare guilt, confusion and unnecessary and often invasive medical procedures. Above all, they insure that your instructions and wishes for the most vulnerable moments in your life will be honored.

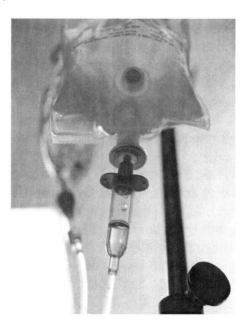

27
I hope they know....the ethical concerns of personhood.

PERSONHOOD IS VIEWED DIFFERENTLY by each society. In Western civilization ethical debates place consideration on the criteria of personhood. Specifically the challenges in our contemporary industrialized society are defining the beginning and the end of human life and the morally relevant boundaries that subject 'a person' to protection. The implications of personhood for patients with any dementing illness and Alzheimer's disease oblige society to make moral decisions to protect these individual's personhood and their rights once they lose the ability to make sound judgments and perform abstract thinking required for consent to their medical and custodial care. How a given society protects a person's rights are the core concerns in the right to life and right to chose, right to die movements. Moral issues are also reflected in the arguments involving embryonic stem cell research, abortion, cloning and even with genetic testing and manipulations with human DNA and cells. There are sociopolitical consequences with our beliefs about life and death.

Personhood or the concept of what makes us a human being in some way assumes a quality of life. This is a central bioethical reflection of ones personal ideal beliefs. Great moral debates will continue over the definition of quality of life. Yet, in American society we support and protect the legal rights of an individual to decide for themselves the extent of their healthcare and the duration and the use of technology to support life in cases where life would otherwise end. In those cases where a person with advanced or end-stage dementia has not left healthcare instructions or preferences and they have no surviving next of kin to make decisions on their behalf, the current law appoints a healthcare guardian to protect their rights and give consent to perform or withhold medical treatments. All patients with end-stage dementia will require others to safeguard their personhood and make best choices regarding their care.

Many people indicate in their living will to forego life-sustaining medical care including the use of feeding tubes, breathing machines and ongoing antibiotic therapy and blood transfusions once they have progressed to an irreversible stage in their disease. This is often the case for end stage heart and lung disease and cancers but also includes the final stage of Alzheimer's disease or a dementing illness. Others may choose to forgo medical treatments at the moderate to severe stage. They choose to pass with dignity, with best care practices and palliative medical care which attends to their pain and other symptoms without prolonging their life or death as soon as they no longer recognize their family or themselves and the life they once lived. The ultimate respect of personhood is following the wishes described by an individual when they can no longer speak or act on their own behalf.

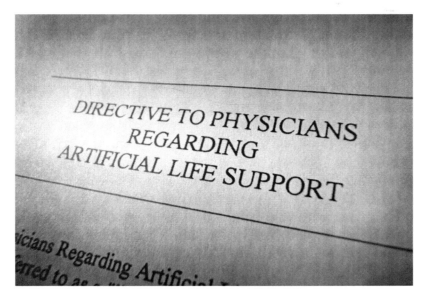

28
I hope they know....the caregiver needs care too.

FATIGUE AND MENTAL EXHAUSTION will reduce a caregiver's efforts. Exhaustion can result in serious mistakes in judgment that can have deleterious effects on both the caregiver and those around them. Caregivers are encouraged to nurture themselves through exercise, proper diet, and adequate sleep. Regular relaxation and stress reduction techniques are extraordinarily beneficial. Meditation is often sited as a good tool for stress reduction, but for some, it requires practice and even coaching in the beginning.

Lots of situations come up in a day demanding attention. It can be difficult to prioritize under these circumstances and you may feel as though you have no control as each demand fights and pushes against the other for attention. One way you can help yourself rise above the confusion and chaos is to breath, in other words, be conscious about breathing. Find a few moments, sit quietly, alone, without distraction, and focus on your breath. That will help you let go of the worries and stress long enough to reconnect with your own life, your own feelings and thoughts. As you inhale, say to yourself *inhale*, and as you exhale, say to yourself *exhale*. Allow the tension in your body to relax. Be aware of your chest as it expands and as your lungs fill with air. Try to hold each breath a few seconds in between. Lie on the ground if this helps, supporting the backs of the knees with a rolled up blanket or towel. Try this for 10 minutes... set an alarm and commit to breathing with this heightened awareness for the entire time. See how you feel when your 10 minutes is up. You should feel revitalized; use this technique to change your perspective, it may help you look for clues which will help you to prioritize your tasks.

Once you have calmed the chaotic thoughts that take over your mind and relax your body, what remains will be a compassionate understanding of what is going on around you. Once you understand this, you can determine what the next step is. As you give care to others, you must give care back to yourself.

Breathing with awareness is a technique I learned in yoga and meditation. Yoga is another great stress reduction technique. Yoga classes can be found just about everywhere these days. You need not belong to a gym, they are offered at yoga centers and also at the YWCA/YMCA. I took my first class at the community Y with my mother when I was 14 years old! There are many more places today and you can begin at your own pace and stay in your own level and choose the kind of class that you enjoy the most. They will also teach breathing techniques. There is no age limit, no body type, no "ideal" to practice this ancient form of relaxation and body toning. You can even get yoga and breathing instruction VCR or DVDs from the public library or supermarkets if you want to start off in your own home. They have shows on public TV and cable shows as well. If you are interested you can find it. The basic yoga postures can help a person to center their thoughts onto their own internal being and leave other thoughts outside. Regular use of breathing techniques, meditation or yoga practice helps alleviate anxiety and has been my stress reduction technique. It works when I practice, and like anything, I have to make the time for it. Aches and pains, even minor injuries have set me back, and I listen to my body and rest. This is good advise for any physical activity.

Another simple technique you can do anywhere is positive visualization. Visualize yourself in settings that make you feel energized, powerful and happy. Using your powers of imagination and creativity are always available to you, 24/7 and anywhere! Finding positive reflections in things that occur outside of you is as simple as a thought. Look around you and find something in your immediate vicinity that once made you smile. Remember that moment and try to replace any negative emotions. These negative thoughts deplete your energy and create mental, emotional, and physical blocks to performing your best. Easily said, but also easily done when you "put your mind to it."

Relaxation with the type of music that calms you down is also very beneficial. Listening to music that you love regardless whether it is vocal or instrumental can promote a sense of calm and well-being. You can listen to your favorite soothing music when you eat, before you sleep, and when you want to relax. Like meditation and yoga, listening to beautiful music can help us maintain our hormonal and emotional balance, especially during periods of stress.

If you are already using these techniques and feel static, or have reached a plateau and anxiety is becoming chronic, then perhaps it is time to try something new. Art therapy and creative writing or journaling therapy suggested in this book for the Alzheimer's patient will have the same positive benefits for the caregivers needs. These creative expression outlets can restore your positive mood. If you mood stays low and you have lost the ability to find joy in anything, and notice your own life patterns have changed, you may be suffering from depression. Check with your doctor.

Make and take time for yourself. It is the best way to become the best caregiver. You are not selfish when you nurture yourself, ultimately you will give more.

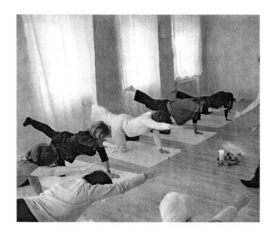

29
Anticipating Grief By Debbi Dickinson

ANTICIPATORY GRIEF IS THE grieving process that begins when we learn that our loved one has a terminal illness. Dr. Therese Rando, a clinical psychologist and well-known authority on grief, states that anticipatory grief is the process where we start to mourn past, present and future losses. When someone has Alzheimer's disease, we mourn the loss of the person he/she was. Sometimes it seems like each day brings another loss to mourn. There is no cure for Alzheimer's and the end result is always death.

The journey you take with a loved one who has Alzheimer's can sometimes take years. In my case, my journey took only two years. It was a short trip but, at the time, it seemed like an eternity. My father, 81, came to live with my husband and I after my mother died suddenly of a heart attack in 1987. He developed Alzheimer's and this is our story.

Dad and I had lots of fun together for the first few years. He joined the Senior Citizen's group in town and I used to accompany him on all the outings—to restaurants, to festivals, shopping trips, and parties. As a family, we went to the movies, Cub games, polo games, zoo, trips to Florida and other destinations. We had three Afghan Hounds who were the joy of his life and we used to take them for walks around the neighborhood together. He had a great sense of humor. Life was great.

Four years passed and we noticed a change beginning to take place with dad. At first we thought it was just "old age." He was forgetting things and began misplacing items, not normal for him. We didn't pay too much attention to it at first. Other behaviors became disturbing and couldn't be ignored. He began rhyming words and thought it was very funny (we didn't) and start laughing.

One day he went for a walk and took longer than usual to return. I went looking for him and found him walking down the middle of a busy street with cars zooming past him. It was winter and his coat was unbuttoned and he had a glazed look on his face. I didn't want to startle him by yelling out to him, so I calmly walked out to meet him in the middle of the street and guided him home. I knew then something was wrong. He was unaware of the danger and said he was just on his way home from the store like other times. He was wondering what I was doing coming to meet him. I said I felt like going for a walk. I felt like crying but I didn't.

When my husband got home from work we decided to make an appointment for him with his general physician. We had to wait a week. The next day my father came downstairs and I stopped him from going outside in his pajamas with a broom. I asked what he was going to do. He wanted to go outside and shovel the driveway before my husband got home work. I thanked him and told him that was thoughtful of him but we'd do it with snow blower later—it would be so much easier. That made sense to him and so he put away the broom.

It was a nightmare of a week. A couple of days later I was on the phone. I turned around and saw him by the stove holding a burning paper towel in one hand. I dropped the phone in the dogs' water dish and stepped over to him and guided him to the sink. We put out the flaming paper towel and luckily he wasn't burned. When asked what he was going to do with it, his reply was that he was going to light the burner.

The doctor's appointment finally arrived. We spoke to the doctor privately and then he examined my father. He referred my father to a neurologist for more tests. Then came the day we were told he had Alzheimer's disease.

I didn't want to believe it. Not MY dad! I was in shock. Of course, now we could see why he was doing what he was doing. Once the shock wore off, I felt depressed because I knew it was only going to get worse.

I grieved for the father I had once known, who was now lost forever. I still loved him and always would, but he was such a different person. He had hallucinations, was paranoid, and didn't make sense most of the time. He was physically declining. His balance became less steady so we got him a cane. When he began falling when we'd be out walking, we had to get him a wheelchair. He hated the wheelchair but he got used to it.

Dad began wandering at night. No longer did he sleep through the night. Our bedrooms were on the second floor. I was afraid he would become disoriented and fall down the stairs since his bathroom was by the stairwell. My husband and I began sleeping in shifts. When my dad would go to bed I would just stay up and work on the computer in the room next to his bathroom. Dad would always get up at 2 or 3 a.m. and see me and ask what I was doing. I would say I was working on a project. Once he went back to bed and fell asleep again, I went to bed. It worked. By then, my husband was up getting ready for work. I would nap during the day when my dad would nap. When my husband got home from work at 5 p.m., I would often go to sleep until he went to bed at 10.

Care giving is a difficult task. What helped was taking breaks. Sometimes my husband would take dad to the movies so I could have some "alone time" or I would go to the Health Club, church, and my weekly Writer's Group meeting. My faith is also what helped me during this time. I'll admit there were times I was angry with God and let Him know it! God was big enough to handle it. Obviously I am still here and didn't get struck down by a bolt of lightening. I prayed a lot and learned to take one day at a time.

Pay attention to your feelings and deal with them in healthy ways. For example, writing in a journal can help you sort through your feelings. If you can't find the words to express yourself, try drawing or painting. The important thing is to find an outlet for what you are going through. A change of scenery can help. Go for a walk. Exercise. Learn to relax—do something fun. There are more resources for help available now than there were when I was caring for my dad. There are many good sites on the internet for support—chat rooms, forums, and message boards. In addition, some communities may have support groups so that you feel you're not so alone. If you think you need counseling, talk to your family doctor for a referral. It's o.k. to ask for help.

In January 1994 Dad fell again and we had to take him to the hospital. He hadn't broken any bones but he was in bad shape. Dad almost died. We never thought we'd be placing dad in a nursing home but after talking to a social worker at the hospital, we decided this was the best thing to do for my dad. It was the hardest decision I ever had to make. We signed the papers and he went straight from the hospital to the nursing home. Dad never came home again.

If you have to place your loved one in a nursing home, know that you did the best you could for as long as you could. I was grateful for the fact that by the time we placed him in the nursing home in February 1994 he didn't know what it was. On his second day there when we went to visit him he thought he was at a restaurant. At other times, he thought it was a hotel. While there, he had an imaginary dog. We visited every day and starting one day, he had a dog now that stayed by his bed. I had to be careful when I went to visit not to step on him. Since I couldn't see him, I didn't know where the dog was! Dad would sometimes yell at me, telling me to "Watch out for the dog. Don't step on him!" Sometimes Dad wanted me to take the dog for a walk...which I did. I didn't argue with him. I tried to keep Dad happy.

He needed help at mealtimes and for all daily routines, called activities of daily living, like dressing and bathing, etc. This seemed to have happened overnight, which did take away the guilt I had felt for our decision for having to place him in a nursing home. I had done a lot for him at home and our roles had become reversed about two years ago. I had felt I the parent and he was the child. There were some occasions where he had even called me "Momma."

He had a room on the top floor, which was the third floor of the facility. As we were leaving, he asked if we were going to go visit mom on the 4th floor. We learned a long time ago not to argue with him, so we said "yes" and we'd tell her he said hi. That made him happy and he smiled and waved goodbye to us from his wheelchair. The elevator doors closed and I started crying. Dad was so out of touch with reality. He'd forgotten mom had died 7 years ago. I was losing dad more every day even though he was physically still with us. I just kept praying he would remember our names and know who we were—and that is one thing he never forgot.

I used to cry because I knew that one day he wouldn't be here. He'd been having various health problems due to his advanced age of 88 and was now in hospice care. Within a couple of weeks we were told to make funeral arrangements for him. He was still alive, but we knew he was dying. I felt helpless. There was nothing I could do to stop what was happening. All we could do was make the most of each day that we had left with him and treasure each moment.

Dad continued to decline and died peacefully in my arms on July 24, 1994.

One's coping strategies vary and are influenced by many factors, such as one's cultural and religious beliefs, the circumstances of the loss, one's relationship to the deceased, previous experiences with loss, support system, and current stresses in one's life. There is no one way to grieve—and no one right way. It will take as long as it takes. Healing doesn't mean you "get over" your loss. It means you remember and move on. The relationship didn't end because he/she died—it just changed. Your loved one will always be a part of you. Find ways to honor your loved one. How we live our life after they are gone is a testament to their love and your love.

Having experienced this journey with your loved one, you can now help others if you choose to and try to make it easier for them as they travel down the rough road of Alzheimer's. Perhaps you may choose to donate to an organization working to find a cure for this devastating disease, or donate books to your local library, or start a website or a support group dedicated to Alzheimer's.

Remember to love yourself and be gentle with yourself.

May the light of love and hope guide you through the night.

30

I hope they know....what services can free up caregiver time.

ALZHEIMER'S PATIENTS CAN BENEFIT from unique services that can help the care giver as well. Adult day care, visiting nurses and homemakers and companions that provide in-home support services on a daily or weekly basis to individuals not in need of medical assistance can be arranged. Some services can include housekeeping, errands, respite care, meal preparation, and social contact. Home health agencies provide healthcare professionals for in-home support services from one to twenty-four hours a day. These professionals include nurses, home health aides, homemakers, therapists, and medical social workers. Reimbursement can be from Medicare, Medicaid, and private insurance.

Another kind of break is respite care in a facility. This kind of care necessitates short-term placement and will need a medical certificate of need or prescription from the doctor. It can help caregivers handle their responsibilities for a few days while alleviating some of the caregiver stress. Continue educating yourself about programs in your area and what special services are available. These programs are there for you!

31
I hope they know....a few thoughts on hope and optimism.

PANDORA 'S BOX TELLS THE story of hope. She had been given a box and instructed by Zeus to keep it closed, but she had also been given the gift of curiosity, and ultimately opened it. When she did, all of the evils of mankind escaped from the box, although Pandora was quick enough to close it again and keep one value inside, Hope.

We have all heard about the power of positive thinking. However, having hope, like optimism means you have strong expectations that things will turn out all right despite bad news, frustrations and setbacks. Having hope has been proven to have a profound effect on your sense of well being and your plan of action and its success. Optimism, a sister to hope, is what allows us to find another antidote to bear life's misery.

When your moral is low, and you are dealing with frustrations and failures, and life's difficulties, it is likely you will feel despair and helplessness. How long you remain in the pessimistic state of mind though can be tempered by hope and optimism. Solutions do exist, and inspiration will come and motivation will follow. Realistic optimism is not the naive yellow smiley face, or the *smile be happy* slogan. Making the choice to be positive is shouldered by hard work and insight. Yes, you have to choose to be optimistic!

Here are some words of hope. Current and best practice information on the treatment and care of patients with Alzheimer's disease will continue to improve. Planning and creating strategies for your unique life circumstance can bring the positive outlook that brings a sense of peace and ongoing optimism about your life. You are giving the best care practices and making a difference for your loved one. It all has a purpose, and you are giving the best you have to offer.

Part III
The Final Journey
As the Disease Progresses

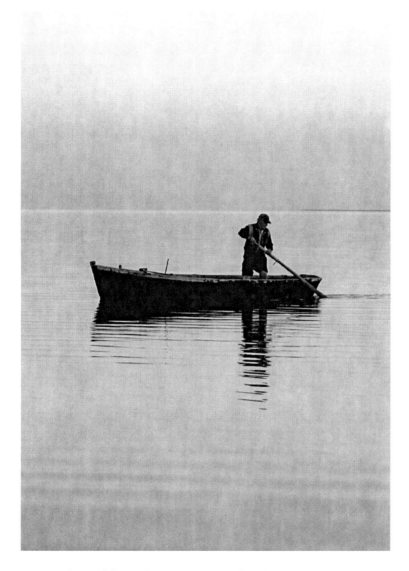

Family and loved ones can make the journey safer.

32
I hope they know....art is in the moment.

Illustrations provided by individuals in The Program of All-Inclusive Care for the Elderly (PACE) at Miami Jewish Hospital and Home, Miami, Florida
Additional interpretive comments by Elizabeth Cockey, Master Art Therapist, Baltimore, Maryland

ALZHEIMER'S AFFLICTED 'ARTISTS' IN art therapy programs are trying to tell us a story using words that don't exist, they know what their images mean, but we don't always. This chasm of understanding is one that Alzheimer's patients face every day. There is a growing effort to use art as a therapeutic tool for those in the grip of Alzheimer's. Art therapy, both appreciating art and making it is often offered in Alzheimer's Day Programs, but much of this work has taken place in nursing homes and hospitals. Yet wherever it is offered, it provides excellent opportunities for patients and their families to connect through art. This modality of therapy has been used for decades as a nonmedical way to help a wide variety of people—abused children, prisoners, cancer patients and now, Alzheimer's patients. It seems to be working, though no one knows exactly how. While extensive research has been conducted on the effects of music and performing arts on brain function—the Institute for Music and Neurologic Function in the Bronx has been studying the phenomenon for over a decade now—there has been comparatively little work done in the visual arts. While the Alzheimer's Association funds studies looking into the quality of life and novel approaches and best practices in care and support, no recent research has been funded by either private or public organizations to explore the benefit of art as a therapeutic modality for Alzheimer's disease that could help standardize its use.

What does exist is anecdotal evidence, while encouraging it remains unclear. For example, we still don't understand why the famous abstract artist Willem de Kooning become more productive, intensely so, as he descended into Alzheimer's? How does frontotemporal dementia, a relatively rare form of non-Alzheimer's brain disease, cause some people who had no previous interest or aptitude for art to develop remarkable artistic talent and drive? Another famous artist with Alzheimer's disease, William Utermohlen created self portraits which were collected and shown in an art exhibition. These portraits chronicle his decent into the disease and how it affected his self perception.

There is still much to learn and understand about the mechanisms of artistic aptitude and expression as the mind begins to unravel. This is one of the areas that could benefit from greater research funding.

In an informal way, doctors like myself, family members and art therapists involved in the art therapy day programs see moderately demented patients recognize and respond energetically to paintings and delight in painting and drawing at a time when they are barely responsive to words. Some patients that are nonverbal most of the time or disoriented and confused can respond dramatically to art group efforts. It appears that recognition of visual art can be very deep, and it does not appear to be just a visual experience, it appears to be an emotional one as well. Caregivers and family alike noted besides improving patients' moods for hours and even days, the art work groups consisting of sculpting and painting efforts seem to demonstrate that the disease, while diminishing sufferers' abilities in so many ways, can also sometimes spark interpretive and expressive powers that had previously lay hidden. An observer can easily detect the focus and concentration on an art project. This kind of focus in many instances is what has been missing in other areas of their lives and activities.

The men and women participants at the Miami Jewish Hospital and Home PACE Alzheimer's Day Program ranged from early to moderate-stage Alzheimer's disease. Each person's diagnostic stage is included with their work. To get more information about the specific stages and the clinical implications, you can refer to the Global Deterioration Scale which describes stages 1-7. These descriptive stages are found in the Appendix.

Introduction to the illustrations

We can take the images that are chaotic or with no sense of an interpersonal world to be representative of the patient's world. It is becoming more and more chaotic as the stages of Alzheimer's progress. The images become increasingly simple; the patient as artist loses the ability to make anything but the most rudimentary shapes. In the later stages, some just managed a round shape when asked to draw a tree or a flower. And there is such a loss of detail that it's difficult to tell what we are looking at. Some could only fill in colors in a coloring book image with no ability to create an image on their own. These changes in the paintings mirror deterioration of specific brain areas. One area vulnerable to Alzheimer's is the parietal cortex, which mediates visuospatial abilities. The paintings reflect this visuospatial disintegration. The paintings become far less cerebral over time and what's left, in the end, is the emotional aspect of the painter. And this emotional quality comes through even in the last paintings.

In particular, the art work that shows the facial details expressed in the "self-portrait" and "lady with a necklace" in the PACE collection were created by one artist with moderate stage disease. They are powerful because there is an emotional content in them. What did I see? What do you see? What does the art therapist see? What is important to note is the ability to communicate emotions through drawing. This communication isn't limited to the professional artist experts. We clearly can see emotion in the facial portrait drawings. This work exemplifies why art therapy can help dementia patient's deal with emotions when cognitive abilities decline. Often behavioral problems result as verbal abilities erode and words fail to express strong feelings. Through art, you can try to maintain a connection between a feeling and how you express it. Choosing vivid colors over dark, making expressive lines or simple lines, these are active, conscious choices.

Art Assignments:

The first images are trees, painted following a request for an autumn tree; the medium was water-based paint on construction paper. Amide Midy, the Activities Coordinator for PACE, demonstrated some photos of a tree in autumn. We discussed trees and leaves and their setting. There were some leaves as well.

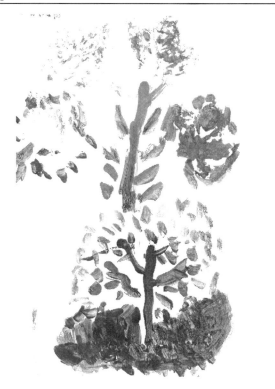

Mrs. Lula Truter, Autumn Tree, Stage 1 Alzheimer's Disease
Interpretation:

Using several colors for her painting, green, blue, yellow and red suggests that Lula is reasonably aware of her reality, using green for the lawn, and several varying autumn colors for the leaves. It might be that she needed some reinforcement to stay on task, denoted by the fact that she drew two trees, one on top of the other. This demonstrates that her ability to understand spatial concepts is diminished; the painting is essentially flat, not two dimensional. On the other hand, it is a happy painting, bright and cheerful. It is possible to see each brushstroke, and if you look closely some of her fingerprints also appear on the page. It seems reasonable that she was concentrating with all her might, attempting to stay on task to complete the assignment.

Mr. Unseul LaFrance, Retired Navy Professional
stage 4, Alzheimer's disease
"I don't want to draw a tree." "My favorite thing"
Interpretation:
I like the fact that Unseul made a conscious decision to paint what he wanted to paint, not what was assigned or suggested. It shows that he is a strong-willed individual who is still determined to make his own choices. Notice that he also signed his name boldly at the bottom of the painting, which communicates to the reader that he counts! The ship he painted is detailed, and looks like it's going somewhere. Interestingly, his choice of hues: contrasting red and blue stripes suggest frustration and restriction within his environment. In spite of the fact that he is in late-stage dementia, I find it remarkable that his attention to detail is still intact. This might be due to the fact that his former experience in the Navy is part of his long-term memory function.

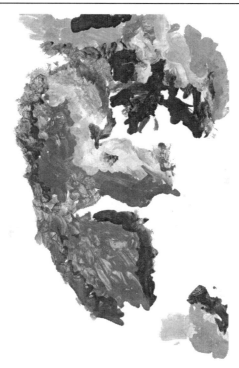

Anonymous artist, Autumn Tree, stage 5 Alzheimer's disease

Interpretation:

The painting by this artist is clearly abstract, not a realistic view of a tree. What this shows is that he is confused and has lost much of his cognitive functioning and the ability to comprehend what's going on around him. Notice how the painting can only be read on one plane. It is flat and without two dimensions. It looks as if he even painted off the page, again indicative that he is having difficulty with spatial concepts. I am struck by a feeling of sadness when I look at this painting. The fingerprints seem to be left behind in the paint by someone who attempting to find his way in a world that is incomprehensible.

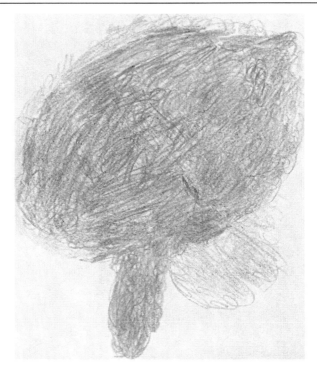

Anonymous, Autumn Tree, stage 4-5, Alzheimer's disease
Interpretation:

This drawing is created by someone with moderate-late stage dementia. Notice the rounded shapes, and very little attention to detail. The shape seems to float in the middle of the page, a rather flat representation, with no middle ground or background. I also notice that the client drew off the page on the right and left sides and towards the top. The translation of images is significantly more problematic for this person, yet the process of drawing can, and will through practice provide an important connection to the world around her or him. Remember that the process of art-making is always more important than the outcome.

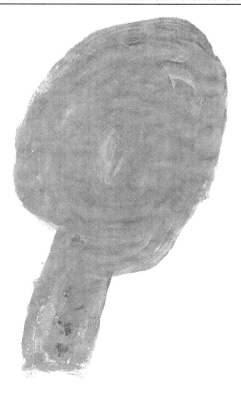

Anonymous, Autumn Tree, stage 5 Alzheimer's disease
Interpretation:

The concept of a tree is apparent in this painting represented by the very strong symbol on the page. I believe the artist is a stoic person, with a strong personality. However, the use of many colors layered one over the other leave behind a muddy ground. I wonder if the artist is depressed. In a couple of areas bright green and red show through, leading me to believe that they were painting from a varied palette, yet unable to articulate. It seems as if the artist painted the same spot over and over and over.

Another Assignment:

On another day we worked with colored pencils and paper and we looked at flowers Here is what we got!

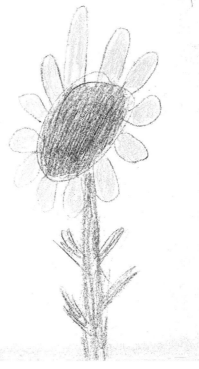

Mr. Enzo Ramerini, Garden Flower, stage 4 Alzheimer's disease

Interpretation:

First Enzo drew the flower in red pencil and then he colored the area in to suggest the middle and outside petals. Despite his mid-late dementia it seems as if he was still able to comprehend a flower and then to reproduce it fairly reliably. What comes to mind for me is "she loves me, she loves me not, she loves me"...and so forth. Flowers are happy symbols and this drawing is uplifting through his choice of color and color combination.

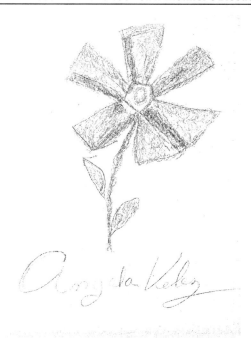

Ms. Angela Velez, Garden Flower, stage 2 Alzheimer's disease

Interpretation:

Angela took her time with this drawing; I can tell this by the attention to detail on the petals, and the fact that she went back over the stem in green. I think that the stem was added last, along with her name at the bottom. But red was her dominant choice of color. She probably started off by sketching in the flower and then adding the stem later. She can still comprehend three dimensions as demonstrated by using blue to fill in one side of each petal on the flower, creating a slight background effect. If you look at the middle of the flower you will see a five sided figure. This indicates a strong desire for order and structure, which may be missing from her experience at this stage in Angela's life. I believe this drawing was important to her, because of the fact that she signed her name in large letters at the bottom, indicating ownership.

And finally, Mr Enzo Ramerini and I hit it off. I drew a picture of a man and then of a woman and asked him to draw his idea of how he looked, and then a portrait of his wife or of a woman. He needed to be reminded of some details of a woman's face. I suggested long hair and a necklace.

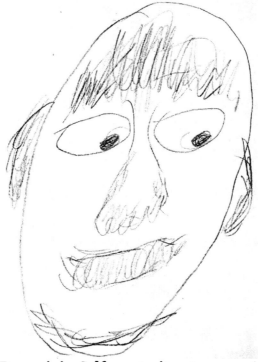

Mr. Enzo Ramerini, Self portrait, stage 4 Alzheimer's Disease

Interpretation:

This drawing reminds me of the portraits young children might create when asked to draw a person. Notice how the head floats in the center of the page and the use of scribbling to indicate the individual's characteristics: nose, hair, ears and teeth. The eyes are looking in one direction, and have a surprised look. I would say that Enzo was happy to do this drawing because of the overwhelming smile that he affixed to the face. The beard may only be indicative; men grow beards, and women have long hair or wear necklaces.

100

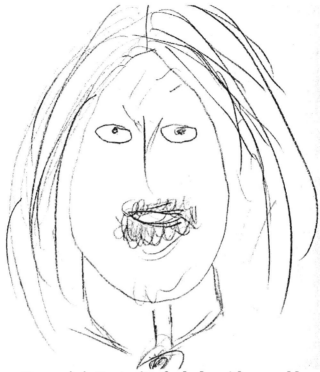

Mr. Enzo Ramerini, Portrait of a lady with a necklace, stage 4, Alzheimer's disease

Interpretation:

I believe Enzo was able to articulate his experience through art the day his wife came to watch as he sketched a portrait of a lady. One can't help but notice how her eyes are staring directly out of the drawing—most likely at Enzo with an intensity and passion that was not apparent in his former drawing of a man. It is likely that her interest in his progress was encouraging to him, as he paid more attention to details.

I believe that the lines going from the bottom of the thin neck and rising up to the sides of the face are her arms, separate from her long hair. Is she also standing with hands on hips? It also seems to me that he feels his wife is, or was beautiful at one time because of the attention to detail with her hairdo.

I think it is interesting to note that even in the later stages of Alzheimer's disease it is possible to communicate with others through the art-making, process. In this case, Enzo's portrait of his wife was meaningful and inspiring to her as well; something they could enjoy doing together.

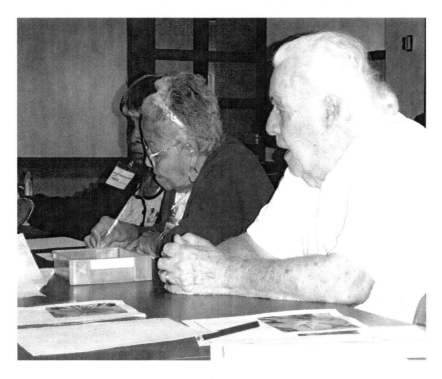

Zoë Lewis©2007 **Art Group at the Miami Jewish Hospital and Home Alzheimer's Day Program, PACE**

Art Projects from the Good Samaritan Nursing Center, Baltimore, Maryland
Also with comments by Elizabeth Cockey, MAT

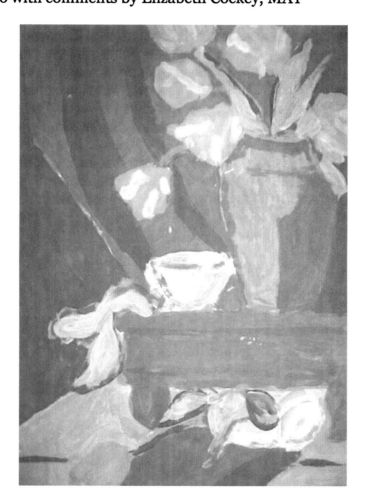

Mrs. D, vase of flowers and tea cup, stage 1 Alzheimer's disease
Interpretation:

Mrs. D. has been a resident at the nursing center for several years, and while she can stand and walk she usually prefers to get around in a wheelchair. She is a delightful and happy person who enjoys dressing up and wearing elaborate jewelry. Mrs. D. loves to tell stories about having a heart attack and being married three times! She loves all things that are colorful and sophisticated and I think nearly all of her paintings reflect her love of color and living life to the fullest.

The painting here is a still life that Mrs. D. copied from an art magazine. She said that the images in the painting, namely the vase of flowers and the cup of tea reminded her of being courted by her late husband. One flower has fallen off to the side and she says that that flower is "love gone bad." When asked about her husbands she simply shrugs and says "I've outlived them all!" Mrs. D. is a passionate person and I think that her choice of color demonstrates having lived a full and eventful life. She is frequently visited by family and friends and it's quite obvious why: she is a delight!

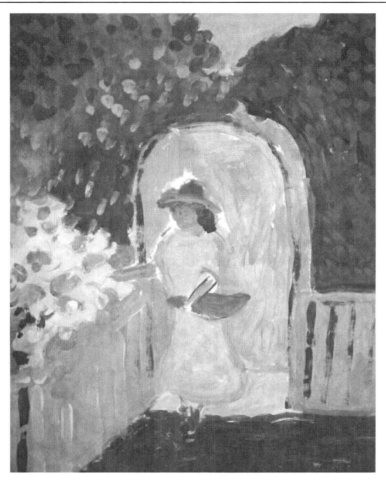

Mrs. S, lady in a garden beside a gate, stage 2 Alzheimer's disease

Interpretation:

Mrs. S. loves to sing, mostly old songs about drinking and gadding about town on Saturday nights. She has been a resident at the nursing center for many years now and has progressed from stage 2—stage 4. But, while she could still hold a brush to paint she was one of the more talented artists, selling her work at the nursing center to staff and visitors. Today, she needs help getting out of bed and sleeps a great deal of the time, but only a couple of years ago she encouraged me to sing while we painted. And, I've been singing during the classes ever since!

The painting Mrs. S. painted is of her earliest memory growing up. She liked to remember the garden out behind her family's home, and how the roses grew in abundance there. Notice how she paints large shapes, using dots or straight lines for the details.

This painting has a background, middle ground and foreground indicating that Mrs. S. still was able to maintain her cognitive functioning during the time she painted this picture, despite what became a steady slide downhill into advanced dementia. And all the while she painted Mrs. S. told stories about living through the depression and WWII. This painting is one of those stories.

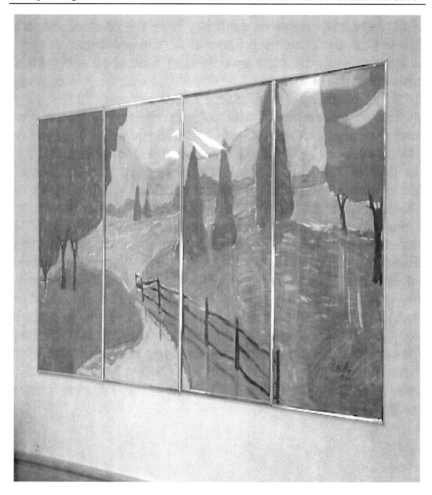

Good Samaritan Nursing Center, framed picture of a landscape mural

Final comments

I am a proponent of working with groups as opposed to one-on-one therapy. The reason for this is because the group setting automatically brings people together. Through this process it is possible to create meaningful and sustainable relationships with people from all walks of life in a multicultural approach. Most of the art therapy groups at Good Samaritan Nursing Center are mixed. In-other-words, I have individuals at all stages of functioning: stage 1 through 5. What happens is that those that can perform with a greater degree of dexterity help the ones who can't. Those who can't use their arms at all are positioned around the outside of the activity table so that they can watch. Nobody is left out.

This mural is 4 feet wide by 10 feet long. Tables were pushed together, and brown postal paper was rolled out over the length of the table. Activity assistants and some of the nurses helped assemble the residents around the outside of the tables, and I sketched in the landscape. Different sections of the mural were outlined in one color or another: dark green for the pine trees and blue for the river. Then everyone was instructed to paint in an area. It took about 2 hours to complete over two separate art therapy sessions and when I hung it up to dry the entire group applauded—their efforts and mine! The reason we painted the spring landscape? It was because none of them could go outside and it was spring. The mural helped ease their emotional pain; most would never walk again, or dress themselves. Painting in this way helped put smiles back on faces of those who would never see home again. The mural was later framed and still hangs in the nursing center today.

Special Acknowledgements

I would like to thank the Good Samaritan Nursing Center in Baltimore for their support and encouragement of my art therapy program. Since the nursing center's inception the main focus has been on creating a better quality of life for the residents living there. How this is accomplished is through recreational therapeutic programs and activities in addition to other recovery modalities such as physical therapy. I have had the opportunity to work for over ten years at the nursing center and am pleased to have a personal relationship with many of the residents, staff and caregivers. Teamwork does make a difference and what we all attempt to accomplish is a better place to live for the residents. *We really are here for good!* I would also like to thank Cesare Tapino, chief administrator and Georgia Martin, director of activities for their input and help in assembling the photos and artwork presented here. And, of course of the residents who do art with me.

33
I hope they know....what are the activities of daily living?

SOME OF THE MORE complex activities of daily living for an adult are the use of the telephone (looking up numbers, dialing, answering, using special calling features), traveling by car or public transportation, food and clothes shopping, meal preparation, housework, medication use (preparing and taking the correct dose), management of money (writing checks, paying bills, evaluating charges and payments) and the general oversight of the home and its security.

Alzheimer's disease and dementia will make these projects and activities more difficult, then impossible. These activities should eventually be taken over by the caregiver. However the list of mechanical activities of daily living that we take for granted after childhood includes bathing, dressing, transferring from the bed or chair, walking, eating, toilet use, and grooming.

As the disease progresses into later stages, these activities will all require assistance. There are clinical tests that the doctor can perform that will indicate the seriousness of decline in these activities. These tests are important because the clinical documentation of decline will determine whether certain services can become available and covered by insurance. Decline also can be used for changing prognosis and also for consideration of long term facility placement care if there is no one to help or provide the assistance safely.

Talk to your doctor about the activities for daily living scales and tests. Also take a moment to secure your assets and put all of your financial papers and documents in order. Passwords and pin numbers need to be recorded and safeguarded. Today with identity theft and computer security risks, preying on the elderly and vulnerable is easier for unscrupulous heartless criminals. Begin to set up fraud protection with your bank and credit card companies and set up accounts that need dual verification for transactions. Early intervention can prevent tragic loss.

34
I hope they know....technology can help.

TECHNOLOGY HAS EMERGED AS a possible solution to meeting the growing needs of an aging population and allowing people with dementia to stay in their own homes for longer. Alzheimer's care assistive technology is a growing field and research and special government and private sector funding is helping to meet the challenges with new and innovative tools and devices to meet the demands in today's world. Yet, dementia can sometimes make people wary of trying new things, adapting to changing situations or learning new skills, so it's important to research products that really suit your situation. To overcome this difficulty, aim to find solutions that can be integrated into the person's normal routine without being noticed, or with the minimum disruption. Remember to respect the individuality of a person when you contemplate using technology, some things will not be a fit, no matter how effective. Involve the person in decisions about which product or solution to use, and take their feelings and opinions to heart. There is a higher chance of success if you can introduce technology when the dementia is still at an early stage, so that the person can gradually get used to the new way of doing things.

Start out with simple. Solutions don't need to be high-tech. Classic "don't forget" ideas that have been used by most everyone are the use of a diary, notebook or notice board that can provide a reminder of appointments, important phone numbers and things to do. Decide on a permanent place to keep important items such as keys and other things that are easily misplaced and write down the locations and keep them on a list on the refrigerator door. Label cupboards, drawers and even rooms to help remember where things are. Label what needs to be labeled. What may seem silly is not for the person walking into a closet thinking it is the bathroom, or putting things away, only to lose them in the wrong place.

Moving into the realm of future technology, soon advances in bioengineering and design targeted for Alzheimer's patients and memory impaired may offer ways to keep persons at home among loving family, within the community, replacing the locked, key-padded floors and wings in the long term care facilities. Tracking and surveillance technology have the potential to address issues of risk management and safety posed by caring for older people with dementia who leave safe environments unaccompanied. In addition, 'smart' technology can reduce risks in the homes of forgetful older people, through the use of sensors to turn off gas burners and running taps.

Finally, memory and communication aids are being developed to support the psychological and social wellbeing of people with dementia that have difficulty communicating. These including touch-screen computer programs, multimedia software to evoke memories and stimulate positive conversation, by incorporating photographs of film stars and songs familiar to older people, and videos about how life used to be.

35
I hope they know....assistive technology exists now.

THE TERM 'ASSISTIVE TECHNOLOGY' refers to any product or service designed to enable people with early dementia illness to remain independent as long as possible. Assistive technology can help people with dementia to retain their self-reliance and confidence. It can also help caregivers monitor the person they are caring for 'remotely'—from another room or another location—without having to watch the person all the time, so they can offer their help when they are needed. They also allow people to choose whether to stay at home for longer or move to a residential home or facility. These technologies include equipment and devices to help people who have problems with:

- memory
- cognition (thought processes and understanding)
- moving about
- speaking
- hearing
- eyesight

Assistive technology ranges from very simple tools, such as walking sticks, or walkers to high-tech solutions such as satellite-based navigation systems to help find someone who has got lost. Selecting the right device is not an easy task; each will require training and practice to some extent. Keep in mind, different people react differently to different products. One person might find a sophisticated monitoring system helpful, while another might prefer a simple tape-recorded message that plays when they open the front door, reminding them to take their keys.

Seek as much advice as possible to ensure a tailored solution for your family situation and needs. There are many different technologies that can be adapted to the needs of someone with dementia and the field is growing with funding and research.

Sensors

Unobtrusive wireless sensors can be placed around the home to raise the alarm if there is a potential problem inside the home of the person with dementia. They are devices which can alert the caregiver or the person with early dementia of impending problems. If the sensors detect possible smoke, gas, flood or fire, they sound an audible alarm as well as alerting a caregiver, key holder or a 24-hour monitoring service. Sensors can be used to detect extreme temperature. A device will send a warning signal if the temperature is very low, very high, or if there is a rapid rise in temperature. For example, this kind of technology can be useful in the kitchen to detect a kettle that has boiled dry or a pan that has boiled over. Devices can monitor ambient temperature by controlling a thermostat that has been raised and left high, or the air conditioner set too low.

- Floods—These detectors can be fitted on skirting boards or floors in the kitchen and bathroom. If the taps have been left running they shut off the water and raise the alarm.
- Scalding baths—A temperature-regulated plug replaces the standard bath plug and changes color from blue to bright pink at high temperatures.
- Carbon monoxide—This alerts caregivers to high levels of carbon monoxide, due to a faulty boiler or gas fire.
- Gas—If someone forgets to turn the gas off, this device will automatically shut off the gas and raise the alarm.
- Falls—Sensors worn on the wrist can detect the impact of a person falling.
- Getting up in the night—A pressure mat sensor is placed by the bed and a sensor activates an alarm

when the person gets up in the night, so that their caregiver can help them get to the toilet.

- Absence from a bed or chair—If a person gets up from their bed or chair and doesn't return for an unusual period of time, or if they don't get up in the morning, this device raises an alarm.

More complex sensor technology can be used for a range of other situations:

- 'Wandering' sensors—If someone likes to come and go inside and outside the house, these sensors, based on passive infra-red technology used in burglar alarms, can help retain their independence. If they don't return to bed safely because they might have fallen, if they don't return home within a pre-determined period of time, or if they are moving around the house outside their normal patterns (such as at night or early am), the sensor will be activated and caregiver help sought.

- Nightlights—Sensors can be set to automatically switch lights on as a person enters or leaves a room. This is useful if someone gets up in the night but doesn't need to be helped by a caregiver.

- Tracking and tagging devices—Tracking devices use satellite technology to help trace someone who is presumed to be or is actually lost. They have their limitations; they are accurate to within certain ranges, feet, yards or miles depending on the geographical area.

- Tagging devices trigger an alarm if the wearer strays outside a defined area. This is controversial as some people consider tagging to be an infringement of a person's civil liberties and personhood, while others believe it maintains it! Personhood and the concepts behind it are discussed in this book elsewhere.

Medication aids

Pharmacies and supermarkets sell pill dispensers, with compartments for particular days of the week and times of day. They help people remember to take their medication at the right time. Automatic pill dispensers are also available. When the medication needs to be taken the dispenser beeps and a small opening permits access to the particular pill at the right time.

Memory aids

Reminder messages are an effective way to remind a person when they enter or leave their home to pick up their keys or lock the front door. These gadgets activate a voice reminding them. The messages can be recorded so that the voice is of someone they know, such as a family member. Messages can also be recorded to remind the person of their daily appointments, to tell them not to go out at night, or to provide reassurance, such as *'Go back to bed, honey— it's night time.'* Door reminders can remind people not to open up to anyone unfamiliar. This can be useful as people with dementia are unfortunately vulnerable to burglary.

Locator devices

These devices can be attached with a key ring or Velcro to items that are often mislaid. If a person wants to find a particular item, they press a color-coded button on a radio transmitter and the device with the corresponding color will beep until the item is picked up.

Clocks and calendars

Automatic calendar clocks can be helpful for people who forget which day it is. Try to find one that shows the date and day of the week too. Clocks that show whether it is evening or morning can help prevent disorientation. This is particularly so in the winter months and after daylight savings time when it is dark before dinner time. Paper calendars which show seasons are also helpful.

Mobility aids and other devices

Other problems associated with dementia include mobility problems, incontinence and difficulties with sight or hearing.

For information about mobility aids, continence devices and pressure relief mattresses and cushions, see your doctor and ask as many of these devices will be covered by medical insurance. Durable medical equipment is also a covered expense by hospice programs.

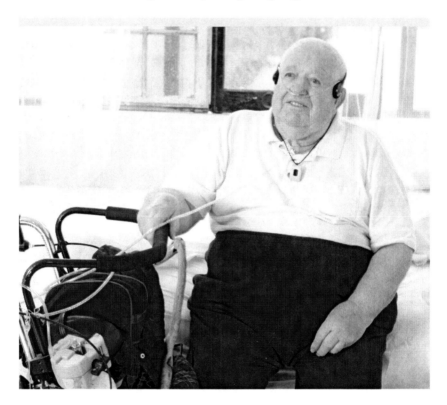

36

I hope they know....why do a swallowing and nutrition evaluation?

SWALLOWING IS A COMPLEX act that involves the coordinated activity of the mouth, pharynx, larynx and esophagus. Aspiration is the passage of food or liquid through the vocal folds into the trachea and lungs. Aspiration is one of the major causes of serious respiratory problems and pneumonia. It is also one of the causes of death for a patient with Alzheimer's disease. The first signs of difficulty with swallowing can be noticed with food pocketing (food held between the teeth and cheek) or choking and coughing or mouth spilling of liquids. A swallowing test will therefore be essential at some point during the disease.

By testing various foods at home, it is possible to determine the effects of food and liquid consistency on swallowing. For example, some patients with poor portion size control will experience less aspiration with thick liquids (e.g., apricot nectar or tomato juice) than with thin liquids (e.g., water or apple juice). There may be many reasons for swallowing difficulties and once it appears there is a change in the ability to handle even small portion sizes and the usual liquids appear to produce coughing or choking, a doctor visit is indicated for a swallowing evaluation.

A swallowing test involves an in-depth feeding and swallowing history, oral peripheral examination, and trial swallows of various food consistencies. A bedside or office evaluation can not rule out silent aspiration. The bedside/office evaluation can be done in the home by a certified speech swallowing specialist if indicated. A video swallowing test may also be needed and this is performed in the hospital and can be arranged by your doctor. If it is determined aspiration is occurring, then the first step may be a simple diet change that would include foods that could be eaten and swallowed safely.

Dietary Modification

Dietary modification is a common treatment approach. Most Alzheimer's patients with significant swallowing difficulties are unable to eat meats or similarly tough foods safely. They require a mechanical soft diet. A pureed diet is recommended for patients who pocket food or who have significant pharyngeal retention of chewed solid foods. Alzheimer's patients vary in their ability to swallow thin and thick liquids. A patient can usually receive adequate oral hydration with thin or thick liquids. Rarely, a patient may be limited to foods with a pudding consistency if thin and thick liquids are freely aspirated. With a modified diet and use of compensatory maneuvers to help with eating, most patients with minimal aspiration can learn, (or with assisted feeding) to maintain sufficient food and drink by mouth to meet nutritional requirements. Full feeding, with the caregiver doing the utensil holding and offering spoon or fork portions, is a feature of end stage Alzheimer's disease.

A nutritionist can also be consulted to make sure that the patient is getting enough nutrients and calories. Sometimes liquid supplements may be needed.

Tube feeding is a method that may be considered to supplement the diet as a last resort if a diet by mouth is not working to maintain the weight of the patient. The decision to tube feed is a difficult one and professionals should be sought. Ask for literature on this topic, there are research studies about the use of tube feeding that you and your doctors can use as a guide. This topic is one which brings enormous emotional reactions if all of the facts and useful information are not made available at the time of decision making. Get information from your doctor or religious body if you have moral or ethical concerns. Education will support your decision.

37
Why the Guilt? By Dr. Patricia Munhall

Caring and the Complexities for the Caretaker of the Person with Alzheimer's

OF ALL THE MYRIAD of conditions that unfortunately affect the aging population Alzheimer's presents one of the most unique challenges for caretakers of persons afflicted with this condition. This I have surmised from various interconnections in my life. As a psychoanalyst I have seen many patients who are caring for a parent or a spouse with this condition and thus have traveled their journeys with them from the beginning of the diagnosis to the end. That is the time when the person afflicted has progressed where they no longer recognize their loved ones, nor can communicate in an authentic way. I also have friends who are or have been caretakers of their parent who has reached this point in the progression of this condition. I have watched patients and friends struggle through the complexities of feelings and emotions that encompass this stage, as I did in the two years prior to my mother's death from Alzheimer's in 2001.

Describing the emotional roller coaster

The path from initial diagnosis where the person is able to converse, recognize, be scared, angry, yet able to love and in particular show love and appreciation to the caretaker is in the course of the disease dramatically altered. The caretaker recognizes this but simultaneously needs to accept their loved one will not be the same person at the onset of the disease then at the end, often when the affected person does not always recognize the caretaker. The person at this stage of Alzheimer's often is not the same person as once known and one can come to the point of asking exactly who is this different person? Of course, it is their mother or father in body, but in mind the person has begun to disappear or metamorphosed into another person.

So the person with this condition is alive in body, recognizable in body, but amazingly gone in so many ways from the caretaker. The person may not always recognize his or her own daughter or spouse. It can be tragic in that the person once known and her personhood have disappeared. The existential self is gone. The spouse or parent once so predictable is now unknown and very unpredictable. So when the self has disappeared, the conscious awareness of self and place, the questions reflecting this state begin. The parent may ask her daughter as she enters her bedroom: *"Who are you?" "Are you new here?" "Who sent you here?" "Are you going to get me out of here?" "I don't want you to touch me."* Or as the person looks at her most beloved grandchild, *"Who is this child?"*

Found walking down the street, the person with Alzheimer's answers to a question, where are you going? *"I am going to meet John"*, the caretaker wonders, "Who is John?" Found in a store, escaping home, a woman fills her pockets with candy, *"I have not eaten in three weeks"* she tells the shopkeeper after having had a full breakfast that morning. *"Leave me alone, I don't want to see you again"* she might repeat a few times a day, every day, to the person who has taken it upon herself to oversee her care and often sacrifice her present day life to do so. The caretaker, tired and exhausted approaches the affected person in an advanced stage of the disease, with a tray for dinner, so carefully prepared and may be aggressively yelled at, *"get out of here; you are trying to poison me."* The challenges go on and on.

Yes, it can be like that. The caretaker needs to know that the person saying such things is not talking for instance to the spouse or daughter, she is speaking from the world of the Alzheimer's condition. Often times it is helpful to remember the former love and I like to believe that the love is still there unable to be expressed.

Sometimes even though the person does not recognize the caretaker, she might not be aggressive or nasty. *"Thank you, you are such a kind person." "That was a wonderful lunch, I am going to tell my daughter about it"*, though you are her daughter! *"What a lovely child"* describing the grandchild.

So it can be a loving person who emerges or it can be a combination. Whatever form it takes, the disorientation, the lack of memory and the ability to recognize loved ones, does elicit profound emotional responses from the caretakers and it is difficult to put a positive spin on it. A sense of humor helps but is severely tested on a day to day basis of caring for your father, who does not know you, accuses you of untrue things, then the next day his mental status changes and he thanks you for caring for him. However the next minute he decides to sneak out of the house, with or without clothes on. Life with a person at this stage of Alzheimer's for the caretaker as was mentioned can become completely unpredictable.

There might even be a day when out of nowhere, the person does recognize the caretaker and hope strikes at the heart of the caretaker. The caretaker says to herself as she looks at her father, *"stay with me, stay a little longer"*. This going in and out of orientation differs for different people, but as the condition progresses it often disappears completely.

The caretaker is now on a rollercoaster of emotions. Anger is a most frequent visitor and most often the caretaker feels guilty about this most appropriate response. Frustration can be a constant companion. Sadness and grief often has the caretaker in tears, in pain, emotionally distraught.

One caretaker said to me: "It is like she is a dead person but still alive at the same time. I mean the person I know, the person I grew up with, who cared for me is gone. I cry so often because I miss her, but she is still with me. Sometimes I think this is far worse than if she had just died. It is a living death"

Another caretaker obviously furious said to me with intense frustration: "I think if she had socialized more with people, or gone out more, just did something more for her mind, she wouldn't have ended up like this. After my father died she isolated herself, and slowly began to deteriorate and now I am left in the position of having to care for her around the clock. The exhaustion is killing me. I will probably die before her."

The circle of life

These are normal thoughts, acceptable; the caretaker is doing probably the most magnanimous act in her life. Is it possible though to have a positive attitude under these circumstances? I will suggest ways in which the management of this condition can be more positive for both the person and the caretaker, mostly through the acceptance of responses. I would like to place emotional responses such as anger, guilt, frustration, sadness, grief and exhaustion in context.

Caretakers who have assumed care of a parent who has reached a progressed state of Alzheimer's need to understand that all feelings they may experience are normal. Here is where a sense of humor might come in to play. Remember your parent had the same feelings about you when you were a toddler. So there is something about a "circle of life" that becomes very magnified with this condition. Today I had two patients with similar thoughts that caused enormous worry, guilt, anxiety and suffering. One of these patients was telling me about her six-month-old daughter:

"I don't know what you are going to think of me, but there are times I am so worried that I am going to hurt her, she starts crying and won't stop, I have been up all night with her and am exhausted. I get so scared that I am going to hurt her, she makes me feel so frustrated that I could pull my hair out."

The other patient was caring for her mother who has advanced stage Alzheimer's:

"There are times I think I might kill her. She was crying and screaming at something she said I did, and I could see myself putting a pillow over her head. I felt so scared and filled with guilt. How could I even have such thoughts?"

Both women were living almost the same lives as caretakers, one of an infant and the other of a mother with advanced Alzheimer's. Their daily chores were more or less the same, feeding, bathing, toileting, insuring safety, but that is where the similarities end. The mother could elicit giggles and cooing from the infant at times and had the knowledge that the path she was on with her infant was ultimately a happy one. The other caretaker was as she later said, "wondering when it would ever end" another thought that produced guilt in her.

Both of these patients' thoughts are completely normal to the context. Caretakers need to be reassured that feeling like you want to do something does not mean doing it*. These are feelings of frustration appropriate to the situation where both women feel powerless. I used to think, now my mother wants me to know how she felt when I was a child. One does such mental machinations during this stage of the condition, wondering just who is in there, who is in this person, who is she, is there a chance she knows what is going on, is she able to think, and we do not have the answers to these questions. At times it all seems like a cruel joke, at other times we know it as a cruel tragedy.

As a psychoanalyst I want to reach out to caretakers and help them express all their feelings, the guilt, the anger, the pain, the grief, the frustration and help them to understand that all these responses are normal. A caretaker is rightfully angry at the situation and for their mental health they need a place to express their feelings. It is not a matter of love; it is a matter of frustration and pain that brings about anger. Never should this lead to guilt.

Thoughts of killing someone might sound strange to be labeled as "normal", but in everyday life in moments of intense frustration ordinary people have these thoughts. It has been documented in the literature that these thoughts are actually common in new mothers and caretakers.

125

Because every once in awhile a tragedy does happen, these thoughts should be evaluated by a mental health professional.

Family Ties

Now there are many caveats to making generalizations. Often times children and parents have had fractious relationships and there are many lingering conflicts that are unresolved. This can produce a different guilt as to waiting too long, or anger that the parent was the cause of the conflict, and once again the caretaker is powerless to do anything about the past. The characteristics of the past are going to influence the caretaker's responses in the present.

This may seem odd at this junction but I think it is important to ask "who is the caretaker?" Literature on caretaker's burn out is abundant and the steps to alleviate the many stresses are described in such literature, whether the caretaker is a family member, a nursing assistant, or even one employed in a nursing home. For the sake of this discussion let us use a daughter as a caretaker. Let us assume that all these emotions are being experienced because the daughter is caring for her mother in her home.

Many times when the diagnosis of Alzheimer's is made the person is living on his or her own. Children living elsewhere have become worried about them because the symptoms of Alzheimer's have become prevalent. Commonly there is one child (now an adult) who assumes more responsibility for the care of the parent for all sorts of reasons, geography, prior relationship, or greatest willingness. There is also an emotional response among all siblings. Thus far we have discussed the more common responses of the main caretaker, but the other family members and the mix engender all sorts of feelings.

The siblings not living in the vicinity feel guilt for that, helplessness over the situation and also the pain and grief of losing a parent who does not know who they are. Often these siblings can rationalize and say well "she doesn't even know me", but depending on the sibling relationships from the past, the ones not present might have added guilt that the responsibility has fallen on to one sibling and thus not doing caretaking, they are further burdened with this guilt. Sometimes the guilt is actually about relief in not being placed in the caretaker's role.

Furthermore the sibling who is doing the caretaking, not only angry at the situation at home, can become angry that the situation has fallen on her, whether her choice or not, may lose her patience with her siblings, all adding to everyone's' guilt and so one can see that the family is at high risk here for everlasting wounds if conflicts are not worked out and feelings processed and talked about with one another.

Another family configuration for caretaking might be the partner of the person with Alzheimer's becomes the caretaker with all the attending emotional responses but felt perhaps in much deeper ways. The situation among siblings may become more or less the same with one sibling doing most of the caretaking of both parents.

So is there an answer, is there a best way, is there a way to avoid the worst of this and preserve the best, which is probably the health of the caretaker and family relationships?

A hypothetical scenario—Family dynamics in care giving.
Even with this hypothetical situation one cannot make generalizations.

The best suggestion I could give under the limitations of a non personal, non individualized, generic recommendation is to read the literature in addition to this book, on caretaking and family dynamics for Alzheimer's patients. You will need to find specific suggestions for your specific situation. There are so many variables, and with that said, with the full acknowledgement of realizing this does not apply to all, but "generally" speaking I present a hypothetical scenario with a few suggestions for caretakers and their families, where the person with advanced Alzheimer's is being cared for by a daughter, one of three siblings. Also because of the generalization here, I am going assume there are no landmines in this family, meaning that this is a loving, generous, giving family.

Some assumptions about guilt

The person who steps up to be the major caretaker needs to understand that no one can care for a person seven days a week, twenty-four hours a day without help. The caretaker needs to take care of herself. She needs periods of time pursuing her own activities and friends. She needs sleep, which might mean hiring an assistant during the night and maybe even during the day. She needs nourishment, food and emotional nourishment. Emotional nourishment is essential to her world of expression. The caretaker needs to express her feelings, positive and negative, to siblings, a partner, friends and perhaps a mental health professional. Emotional responses must be vented, never repressed. This might be the most important aspect as to the health of the caretaker.

Actually, from my professional and personal experience, a critical evaluation needs to be done by the entire family as to whether the person with Alzheimer's should be cared for in anyone's home. There usually is a time when this is feasible, where the person's dignity and safety can still be maintained. I would tentatively suggest when the person becomes disoriented and does not recognize people around her, on the grounds of her own safety, dignity and with the entire quality of life question, that the family come together to consider an assisted living or nursing care facility.

Interestingly enough this is often the juncture where the most guilt sets in. Nothing seems worse then placing a loved one in a care facility. Caretakers and other family members may see it as giving up. It is relinquishing responsibility. It is missing the person. It may and realistically so, be the final resignation of the inevitable. For many, this is the most difficult decision to be made. Symbolically what also may be occurring, especially if the other parent is not alive, is the dissolution of the family home. Then there is more grief and sadness. There is more anger as well as the guilt.

The anger might also intensify, now for additional reasons. Even at the best of nursing care facilities, you may walk into her room at the wrong time and see your mother not being treated the way you would like her to be. You also see her among other people with the same or similar conditions and wish you could take her away from this setting. Some siblings or friends may not come to visit very often if they find that the affected person does not recognize them. This could infuriate the primary caregiver who is still routinely visiting the mother. The caretaker might feel abandoned.

Guilt at this stage comes in different forms. The caretaker might feel guilt in that she did not try hard enough and ruminates that she could have kept her mother home longer with additional effort. Another form of guilt actually comes from feeling relieved that she no longer has to care around the clock for her mother. The siblings might also feel this guilt of relief because the caretaker is no longer the one making the most sacrifices. Once again these are all normal reactions, not to be thought of in a critical way.

As with most conditions where individuals eventually come to live in a nursing care facility at this stage of life there are so many emotional responses to cope with for the caretaker and for the siblings. One mentioned is the loss of "home" as once known, often taken for granted, and now solely missed.

With Alzheimer's patients, questions of authentic living are asked. Does a family travel for eight hours to visit a mother who does not recognize them? What is important here is that family members do come together and that effort is made to stay together during this difficult time. New rituals need to be created and in an ideal situation they do include visits to the mother.

I remember how sad I thought it was when I visited my mother in one such facility and witnessed all the abandoned older people. There were so few visitors, Mother's Day, particularly stands out. Some questions cannot be answered. We do not know what is going on in the minds of patients with Alzheimer's, but I do know they know when they have a visitor. So even if they do not know who you are (and can we be sure?) most seem pleased to have company. Knowing that you have made your mother happy in her own way can help with your own emotional responses. You know you have done a good action for her. This is positive. To make your mother happy, this is wonderful.

To make your loved one happy whether she knows you or not, is a wonderful return of selfless love.

38

I hope they know....to reassess the patient and family goals of care often.

A CAREGIVER CAN BE any family member, a son, daughter, grandchild, nephew, or a spouse. They can even be a more distant relative or a close friend or a fee- for-service professional. Anyone can develop a sense of burden in caring for a dementia patient. The duty to ensure the safety of someone with moderate or later stage Alzheimer's disease can become overwhelming.

The person who is the major caretaker needs to understand that no one can care for a person seven days a week, twenty-four hours a day without help. As I have stressed in other chapters, the caretaker needs to take care of themselves as well. They need periods of time to relax with their own activities and friends. They need restful sleep, nourishment, and emotional connections with other healthy individuals. When these aspects of balanced life are deprived, the health of the caretaker suffers.

There is no simple test that can determine if you are suffering from "caregiver burnout". However, it is often obvious to you or others. There is a modified caregiver burnout test in the Appendix. Take the test now and frequently to assess changes in your attitude. Ideally the family and patient goals of care should be assessed continuously, but certainly well before moderate to severe caregiver burnout occurs. Try using this test frequently and review the results with your family, other caregivers and doctor.

The test is adapted from an original article published in Gerontologist and is used to assess burden in the relatives of impaired elderly, but it is also an excellent tool for determining burden for the Alzheimer's patient caregiver.

39
GRATITUDE

I HEAR MY BREATH
I feel your breath
our heart beats are integrated
in the rhythm of life.
I have gratitude for being alive
for sharing with you
a unique, universal connection.

Now, I remember
my first breath
meal
step
word
relationship
kiss
vision
project
meditation
my first conscious connection with Qi,
with Om,
with You.

None of them can be taken for granted
today.
Each one, every time they are repeated,
are like a first time again.
As sacred, as beautiful, and as unique.
What keeps me fully alive,
in gratitude,
is to cherish every moment,
every step I take as a gift

to bring more consciousness
within my actions, thoughts,
integration within the creation,
and with everyone around me.
Thank you dear parents
for your union, love,
that allowed my conception.
Thank you, mother,
for creating space
for my first heart beat
that guided me within my body.
Thank you, dear lover,
awaken with me
harmony and vision
Thank you, dear friend,
for being part of my life.
Thank you, dear family,
For sharing ups and down
for always being there for me.
Thank you, Creation,
for nurturing me.
Thank you, community,
for supporting me.
Gratitude is the Greatest Gift.

By Christelle Chopard, 2007
http://www.dharmi.com

40
I hope they know....when to recognize major behavioral symptoms.

REMEMBER THAT A PERSON with dementia is more easily agitated because the brain has physically changed and no longer functions in a healthy manner. The specific syndromes of agitation, including delirium, psychosis, depression, anxiety, insomnia, sun downing, (the early evening-dusk agitation bursts), aggression and anger, and pain, are the major behavioral symptoms common to dementia illnesses and Alzheimer's disease. Families are often surprised by how angry or guilty they feel when they lose patience with their loved one. Here is a list of common behavioral symptoms:

- Irritability
- Frustration
- Excessive anger
- Blow-ups out of all proportion to the cause
- Constant demands for attention and reassurance
- Repetitive questions, demands, or telephone calls
- Stubborn refusal to do things or go places
- Constant pacing, searching, rummaging
- Yelling, screaming, cursing, threats
- Hitting, biting, kicking

The main problems that cause agitation are new or existing physical and medical problems, environmental stresses, sleep problems, and underlying psychiatric syndromes of depression coexisting with anxiety. Agitation can be treated in a number of ways. You and your doctor will explore what can help an agitated person.

Here is a short list of covered topics for managing agitation in this book:

- Providing the right environment
- Supervising activities and using assistive technologies
- Learning how to talk with a person who has dementia
- Getting support for families and caregivers and improving coping skills
- Medications
- Music for comfort
- Gentle touch for comfort
- Art therapy
- Life review and journaling

Remember it is the disease, not the person acting out.

41

I hope they know....what to do for inappropriate sexual behavior.

THE NUMBERS OF PEOPLE with Alzheimer's disease and other types of dementia who exhibit inappropriate sexual behavior are reportedly small but because research into sexuality and dementia is limited, estimating the actual number of people whose sexual behavior affects the life of their caregivers is difficult to judge. A lot of inappropriate and aggressive sexual behavior seen in people with Alzheimer's is observed in the later states of the disease and is often a real problem for the caregivers in the long-term care facilities, but it can occur at any stage. It can be a cause of embarrassment for the family or even lead to further social isolation of the person with Alzheimer's disease and his or her family. One of the most important things to remember is that people with dementia are as entitled to express their sexuality as anyone. However, as the severity of dementia symptoms increase, there will come a time when the person is no longer considered to be acting with full understanding of the consequences of their sexual behavior.

What is sexually inappropriate behavior?
- Public masturbation
- Making lewd remarks and advances
- Touching others or oneself inappropriately
- Conversation that is overly sexually charged

Most people with Alzheimer's disease lose sexual drive as the disease progresses. This can also be a result of other causes, like medications, or hormonal imbalances. Most inappropriate sexual behavior exhibited by people with

Alzheimer's is unwanted sexual advances such as touching, lewd remarks or public masturbation. It appears more often in men. Sometimes inappropriate sexual behavior combines with aggression and can create a much more serious problem. These kinds of aggressive problems can be very difficult to manage especially when the caregiver is an older spouse or when the events occur in public or in the home or long term care facility where sexual 'abuse' or other violations may be misunderstood and reported by the observers, staff or caregivers. In a small number of cases these kinds of inappropriate sexual behavior can be of a serious nature. Sometimes problems occur simply because the person with Alzheimer's disease is much bigger and stronger than their caregiver. If the inappropriate sexual behavior becomes violent and persistent and creates a threat, and the person with Alzheimer's does not respond to verbal instruction to stop, then the physician must be contacted. Often there are possible medication adjustments or other medical interventions that may be needed. Do not think this behavior will pass, it may not simply go away and steps need to be taken for safety.

Dealing with inappropriate sexual behavior in Alzheimer's

In most cases this behavior is easy to deal with. A kind firm instruction to stop often works. If the person cannot be redirected, then taking the person to a different room for some privacy to masturbate may be a solution. Dealing with sexually inappropriate behavior often requires different approaches at different times. Each person is unique. There are a number of strategies that you can try.

- Use a gentle or kind instruction to stop. Use humor if it seems appropriate. Try not to sound demanding or angry as this often can aggravate the situation, cause shame or anger.
- Try using different instructions if they do not respond to being asked to stop. Use simple sentences. "Do not touch your penis." "Take your hands off of my leg", "Do not touch there."

- Try redirecting the person to another activity, give them something else to think of or do.
- Look at their day to day activities and try to offer a program that includes more physical activities.
- Offer movement if they are able to ambulate or exercise.
- Do not use physical force to move or push away unless you believe you are in danger.
- In an emergency you must call for assistance either from a relative or from the police if you consider that you are in danger.
- Make sure the environment is safe. Keep all areas of the home safe, with good visibility.
- Never have weapons in the house.
- You need to involve your doctor and caseworkers that can offer support, help and advice.
- Medications are available that can be used short term to assist when sexual behavior is of an aggressive nature.

Remember, it is the disease and not the person making the behaviors.

42
I hope they know....how to interpret nonverbal communication.

PATIENTS IN THE LAST phase of Alzheimer's disease begin to lose their ability to form meaningful sentences and may only repeat words with little or no meaning. Communication difficulties in patients with Alzheimer's disease are a major source of caregiver strain because of the psychological and interpersonal burden they present.

Understanding the patient with advanced Alzheimer's requires a fundamental transformation in our communication habits. This is "learning how to talk with a dementia patient." There is a section on learning how to talk in this book. There is also a need of reorientation towards attentive observance of nonverbal signals. Those who have parented an infant have developed similar skills.

Nonverbal communication is the process of sending and receiving wordless messages using body language, facial expressions, posture, eye contact, and sounds. Caregivers can interpret these messages and distinguish them from unconscious communication which may be verbal outbursts or words that have no meaning. This is a challenge, but consistent care giving will develop this skill. The basic human needs of hunger, thirst and toileting will require assistance without the patient requesting it. These needs may be expressed with non verbal messages, like position shifting, fidgeting, facial grimacing and other examples. Establishing routines for nutrition and toileting can enhance the quality of life, reduce tensions and problematic behaviors and help caregivers. These areas are discussed elsewhere in this book as well.

Keep in mind your own nonverbal messages. For the caregiver, maintaining a non-judgmental facial expression, relaxed body and an even tone of voice are important and if you are stressed, very difficult to retain. Try to remind yourself that you are in control and allow compassion and empathy to guide your responses.

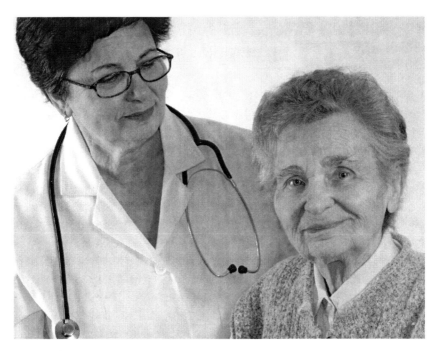

43

I hope they know....nonverbal signs of pain and discomfort.

PHYSICAL PAIN AND EMOTIONAL discomfort are commonly experienced by people with dementia. In the later stages the person is less able to complain about the specifics that hurt or bother them. Instead, they may act out and get angry or aggressive, hit or scratch or show other behaviors not normally associated with the expression of pain or discomfort. In fact, often persons with difficult behaviors may actually be expressing pain, discomfort or emotional discomfort.

Pain may be caused by many things and often is from infections, inflammation or constipation. The source of pain needs to be evaluated promptly. Emotional discomfort may arise from unpleasant memories, anxiety regarding something present at the moment and from the disease process itself. Discomfort may come from environmental sources or from less aggravating internal causes. Distinguishing between causes of pain and discomfort in a nonverbal patient is difficult and professional care should be sought. Here is a list of a few of the signs of pain and discomfort used by medical care professionals.

- Facial expressions: Grimacing, frowning, blinking, tightly closed or widely open eyes, frightened, weepy, worried, sad

- Moods: Irritability, confusion, withdrawal, agitation, aggressiveness

- Body language: Tense, wringing hands, clenched fists, restless, rubbing/holding a body part, hyper- or hypoactive reflexes, guarding a body part, noisy breathing

- Voice: Moaning, mumbling, chanting, grunting, whining, calling out, screaming, crying, verbally aggressive

- Behavior: change in appetite, sleep mobility, gait, function, participation, exiting, wandering, elopement, physically aggressive, socially inappropriate or disruptive, resists cares.

The assessment and treatment of pain and discomfort in dementia patients is best accomplished by medical professionals. If you are managing someone at home, try to keep a diary of what you observe and when you observe it, notating observations like onset, duration and what if anything made it better, then go over it with your doctor or visiting nurse. Uncontrolled pain can be the cause of suffering and this can be treated.

44
I hope they know....what are environmental stressors?

PEOPLE WITH DEMENTIA ARE very sensitive to the environment they live in and are more likely to get agitated with "environmental stresses" or from things surrounding them that affect their lives. They are less able to handle changes, uncertainty and other situations that they could manage when they were well. The ideal environment for a person with dementia provides clear, calm, and comforting structures. Changes in the home may need to be made and often this is not an easy situation to arrange. Routine is very important, since changes in schedule or rushing can cause extreme disappointment, frustration, or fear. A physically comfortable environment is important. Noisy, poorly lit, or improperly heated areas can cause increased agitation. If you are adding assistive technologies, these can initially cause some tension as well. Mood can be affected as easily as modulating lights sources. Keeping areas well lit with modulating devices just one of many positive strategies.

Providing the Right Environment

It is important to evaluate the person's environment. Think about his or her bedroom, and daytime areas. Think about their schedule to see if any thing may be contributing to agitation. Some individuals become particularly agitated at specific times of the day. Try to observe and listen or see what they might, that you overlook every day. It may help to change the person's routine to avoid these problems. It is helpful to try to do things in the same place at the same time each day.

Agitation may result from thirst or hunger. If a person with dementia forgets to eat, maybe they forgot where the kitchen is. Offer frequent snacks and beverages. It takes a bit of a detective mentality, but observation and notation can help discover distressing patterns which can then be eliminated or adjusted.

Research is ongoing in a new area called neuroarchitecture, where the goal to mood-alter and mood-boost certain brain processes using interior design, décor and lighting is the focus. More information can be obtained from the Academy of Neuroscience for Architecture, (ANFA) on their recent developments.

Private companies also specialize to improve home and nursing facility environments. Improving psychological well-being using the mix of art and science, John Zeisel, PhD, of Hearthstone Alzheimer Care, Woburn Massachusetts has a company dedicated among other things, to design therapeutic environments for dementia sufferers. His company also does research with top designers to help modify the home looking at factors like lighting, interiors, room layouts and space. In 1990 the American Association of Retired Persons (AARP) published his consumer guide—*Selecting Retirement Housing.*

It is optimistic that these changes could be made available soon for everyone, but new frontiers in care will rapidly change how we live in the future and strategies will someday be affordable for all.

45

I hope they know....learn to talk with a person with Alzheimer's disease.

THE FOLLOWING SUGGESTIONS CAN help you communicate more effectively with a person who has dementia. You can "learn to talk" with a person with dementia if you keep in mind a few thoughts. People with dementia often find it hard to remember the meaning of words that you are using. They may have trouble to think of the words they want to say. You may both become frustrated, and you may feel angry; but showing your anger can create anxiety and then an agitation cycle. If you are about to lose your temper, try "counting to ten," or take a few deep breaths and be conscious of your own emotions, remembering that the person has a disease and is not deliberately trying to make things difficult for you. Again, compassion will always be helpful. Here are the basics.

Try not to insist on facts. For example, if the person with dementia is mistakenly convinced you didn't see her yesterday, then focus on her feelings of insecurity today. "I won't forget you," is the message you need to send. Try to talk about feelings rather than arguing over facts. If a subject of conversation makes a person more agitated or frustrated, it may help more if you drop the issue rather than keep on trying to correct a specific misunderstanding. He or she will probably forget the issue and be able to relax in a short while. Don't assume anything, try to gently gauge the depth of need and proceed slowly in conversations.

Always identify yourself by name and call the person by name. The person with more advanced Alzheimer's may not always remember who you are; don't keep asking, "Don't you remember me Mom?" These kinds of questions may provoke anxiety or sadness. Always try to approach the person slowly from the front and give him or her time to get used to your presence, and then initiate conversation. Maintain eye contact while you speak. A gentle touch may help, but put this technique into your own personal context with the person if you use it for comfort or calming. Try to talk in a quiet place without too much background noise such as a loud television or other people in a nearby conversation. Speak slowly and distinctly. Use familiar words and short sentences and try to keep things positive.

In activities and choice making, offer few choices with affirmative actions like "Let's go out now," or "Would you like to wear your dress or pants today?" Keep it simple if frustration is apparent.

If the person seems angry or upset and you don't know what he or she wants, try to ask simple questions that can be answered with yes or no or one-word answers. Use gestures, visual cues, and verbal prompts to help. For example, if you suggested a car trip, then get out the coats, get the car keys and open the door, and say "Let's go for a drive now."

Take the time, be patient and above all remember you can control your feelings.

Empathy comes from within your heart, try to remember they have a disease and are not able to process a logical or emotional behavior as once they could.

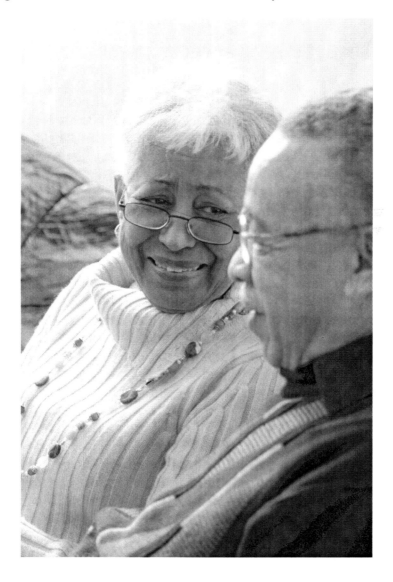

46
I hope they know....music can be used for comfort.

ALZHEIMER'S RESEARCHERS CONTINUE TO seek alternative healing methods beyond medication and conventional therapy. Music therapy has been studied extensively and now is used as a treatment method for Alzheimer's patients despite that it will not provide a cure. Research studies show that the use of music therapy can boost mood, improve sleep and increase levels of hormones, including melatonin, that promote a sense of well-being, thereby improving the quality of life in Alzheimer patients. Music is a medium of expression which can be used to reach patients experiencing a lost willingness and ability to interact with family members or caregivers. Music can substitute as a communication device, instead of words for the patient who has difficulty with language. It is found that singing songs from a patient's childhood or early adulthood will access their long-term memory and promote social interaction with other participants and family members. To that end, more and more nursing homes, day programs and hospices are finding that working with a music therapist to help create an individualized music therapy intervention can make a big difference in quality of life for the dementia patient. Music therapists can teach you to use music to calm and engage a person when they are upset or to bring joy for the sake of joy.

Here are some suggestions. Sing or play familiar songs from the era and culture that correspond to the person. Keep in mind the culture roots of an individual, as not all music will be beneficial if it was not a part of their early life, not every childhood song in your repertoire corresponds to a particular person, including other family members or even your spouse. For this reason, a music therapist can help family and caregivers make appropriate individualized music selections. Music can be used instead of medications and help with mood stabilization, calm an agitated patient, or even bring on sleep and improve appetite.

There are many evidence-based studies which also show that individualized music listening can be used to calm agitation in nursing facility residents with dementia instead of resorting to restraints and medications which sedate. I have personally worked with hospice patients using individualized music therapy and the positive benefits were observed by staff and family alike. Music should be part of the care you give to a dementia patient, but it can also be used by the caregiver for relaxation and mood improvement. In other words, music is a blessing for us all.

The American Music Therapy Association can give greater detailed information and provide resources about ongoing international research studies in the use of music therapy in Alzheimer's disease and dementia illnesses.

47
Music and Alzheimer's Disease
By Dr. Suzanne B. Hanser, EdD, MT-BC

I hope they know music can be appreciated at any stage, at any age.

PEOPLE WHO HAVE DEMENTIA live in the moment. They cannot count on remembering the recent past; they cannot plan ahead reliably. But they can invite others to be present with them in the moment. When they do, it is important to respect what comes up in that moment, even if they are confused or agitated. Acknowledging their feelings of frustration and redirecting their attention to something pleasant may be just what the doctor ordered. Listening to music can draw their interest naturally to a familiar and comforting source. Regardless of the stage of disease, everyone can participate in listening, tapping a foot, singing, dancing, drumming along, or reminiscing about a favorite piece of music.

Music is something that everyone is exposed to early in life. When the mother's voice or lullaby is paired with love and sustenance, her sounds will carry deep meaning for the child. As the child grows into adolescence and adulthood, music that is popular at a special dance, played during a spiritual, religious service, or sung at a holiday or celebration, will evoke deep feelings. Later in life, the music that is linked to these significant memories still will be appreciated, whether or not the listener has developed dementia. This is because that well-known music is hardwired firmly into the part of the brain known as the hippocampus, the container for long-term memories. If the music also stirs up strong emotions, it will simultaneously activate another part of the brain, called the amygdala. The amygdala is the seat of emotions, and like the hippocampus, is accessed immediately and directly. So, even when the thinking part of the brain's cortex is damaged, music goes right to the amygdala and hippocampus, without requiring the person to think about it. The listener does not have to make a conscious connection with the music to experience the joy or sorrow associated with it.

Rhythm is basic to our heartbeat, the circulation of our bloodstream, and the way we walk and talk. A strong, rhythmic beat demands attention from the listener, and provides a clear structure for exercising or walking. Rhythmic music instructs the listener to move at a certain time without requiring any spoken directions. It also invigorates the listener like a newly charged battery. Music that gets faster and faster will result in gently persuading the person to move faster and faster. In the same way, music that slows down gradually may help a person calm down and relax. But, it is not quite that simple. The music has to hold significance for the listeners in order to influence their behavior.

The sense of rhythm is with us throughout our lives, and is one of the functions that is maintained until near the end of life. For this reason, it is possible for people in the late stage of dementia to be able to keep time with music, and to move with the beat of a well-known song. Rhythmic music is often peppy and can lighten up the atmosphere, gently prompting listeners to look around and pay attention to their surroundings.

The rhythm makes music a highly structured, continuous activity that keeps on going, measure after measure. Even when individuals with dementia fail to process a particular note or musical phrase, the rhythmic beat will occur at a predictable time, and they can pick up the music when they are focused and ready.

While caregivers and family members are playing music that holds lasting memories for the person they care for, they can expect to see recognition, a change in mood, and perhaps delight! Identifying the most meaningful music is the hardest part of this assignment, but well worth the effort, to create an experience of high quality that is appreciated by all. Consider making music listening an integral part of the daily schedule. Encourage singing and dancing along. Talking about the music and the memories it elicits may also be an enjoyable, shared experience. Find some percussion instruments, and make your music listening experience a party. If the person you care for has played musical instruments or enjoyed singing earlier in life, get hold of some instruments and familiar music. Start a sing-along and invite others to join in. Musical abilities are often amazingly preserved. It usually requires someone to start off with the first verse, and those well-rehearsed musical skills come right back.

I hope they know that music can focus attention and foster self-awareness.

It is not possible to close the ears to sound, and sounds are everywhere. Too much sound and background noise can be over-stimulating and downright annoying. Sounds that come as a surprise can be frightening. Sounds that are loud can be distracting to concentration. Even soft sounds can be unsettling when they are unwelcome. So, it is understandable that people with dementia may become quite agitated when their senses are overloaded with sound. Because it is harder for them to concentrate, any sound can be perceived as noise, and noise is always irritating or disturbing. Of course, it is necessary to pay close attention to sounds in order to make meaning of them. The person with dementia may have difficulty deciphering and comprehending spoken words because the brain is not processing them fully or because there are too many distractions. But when the sound is music, the message is nonverbal, and this communication does not require the same formal means of understanding.

Background music is pleasant for some, but in most cases, it is a source of confusion for the person with dementia. This is why it is essential to put music in the foreground and use it for a specific purpose. Initiate a musical activity when there are no other demands made on the person. If the goal is to focus attention, engage the individual with dementia in humming, singing, or playing instruments that are easy to master. Give one instruction at a time, keep a simple beat or repetitive pattern, and start with a single phrase. Rain sticks, drums and shakers can enhance the musical effect while focusing the attention of the player, but make sure that the overall sound is pleasing. After contributing to the musical creation, the music-maker is bound to feel a sense of competence and confidence, often sadly lacking in the person who is losing mental abilities. Better yet, consult with a music therapist to conduct a formal assessment and recommend a program to help meet achievable goals.

I hope they know that music brings back sweet memories.

When the person you care for is impatient, frustrated, or angry, there is a way for you both to reduce stress. First, find several pieces of music that are familiar and meaningful. Think about the music that was popular when the person with dementia was a young adult. Research the music that was played at a prom or wedding, or associated with the culture or religion of the person. Select a piece that grabs the attention with strong or syncopated rhythms, catchy lyrics, or memories of exciting times. Play the music and move or dance around, encouraging the person with dementia to follow you. Use this physical release of energy to replace body tension, letting the music guide the movements. Make sure that the music is not too fast or complicated, or it could result in more agitation. Use your judgment to determine if it is advisable to play the piece again, or move on to something different. When you introduce another piece, choose some music that is softer, slower, has longer phrases, or more flowing melodies. While this music plays, give yourself a gentle facial massage, and encourage the person with dementia to do the same. If you are caring for a loved one and feel comfortable,

153

use gentle touch to massage your loved one's tight muscles. Next, circle your head around your neck, slowly and comfortably, working out any tension in the neck. Move your shoulders in circles, and delicately guide the person you care for to imitate you. Stretch out arms and legs, bending them gently, without effort. Help the person with dementia to move with you, in an attempt to bring relief to taut muscles throughout the body.

Identify a piece that the person with dementia loves. Play this as a finale to the medley of beautiful music, and sit back and enjoy. If feasible, talk about the music, the memories it evokes, and reminisce about wonderful times.

I hope they know music can help start the day.

Sometimes it is just too hard to get out of bed and start a new day. Especially in winter, and when the weather is inclement, an external source of motivation may be necessary to jumpstart getting going. Playing music that is associated with festive times, happy feelings, and fabulous memories is a great way to approach the day ahead. Energetic music is capable of arousing the senses and waking up the mind. It is also able to stimulate heart rate and enhance mood. So, putting on music that means something to the person with dementia can have positive impact, cognitively, psychologically, and physiologically.

Humming, whistling and singing are welcome accompaniments to the ablutions that begin the morning routine. These active means of generating one's own music are particularly effective in augmenting brain activity and boosting the brain's release of chemicals that trigger the flow of energy and pleasure. This process can heighten self-awareness as well as interest in others and the surrounding environment.

All of this is helpful in enhancing mental acuity. However, lasting change is hard to come by when the brain's neurons are not firing consistently to sequence thoughts and behaviors. Even though socialization is a desirable action, conversation may be difficult for the person with dementia to follow. Interactions with caregivers and others are strained when the person repeats certain phrases over and over, or has trouble sitting still. In contrast, dancing, singing, and music-making engage people together and leave room for any level of participation. Everyone may listen passively to music or be inspired to create their own. They may accompany the music that is playing or sing their own solos. No talent is necessary to respond to music and let it bring out the positive and creative within.

I hope they know music can help end the day.

"Music hath charms to soothe the savage breast, to soften rocks, or bend a knotted oak," or so William Congreve would have us believe, when he penned his play, "The Mourning Bride," in the 1600's. While there is no scientific evidence to this effect, there is considerable research on the palliative qualities of music. Listening to music that spurs peaceful associations, stirs comforting memories, or incites calming images is capable of relaxing people deeply. Some experiments have shown that certain restful music can even put people into an altered state of consciousness.

No matter what the level of neurological impairment, almost anyone who can hear music is affected by it. So, when the sun is descending in the sky, and sundowning causes people with dementia to become uncomfortable or anxious, participating in musical activities can change their dispositions and transform their temperaments. Listening to familiar music initiates a positive frame of mind when recognition of that music and its comforting associations are brought into consciousness. But much more effective is the actual creation of sound and music that engages many parts of the brain at once, and redirects attention from the unpredictable perceptions at this challenging time of day to the sounds that access a lovely, long-term memory.

This familiarity breeds contentment in a confusing world. It enables the person who cannot depend on recent history to recede temporarily into an era that resides in past memories that are safely stored away. Music elicits thoughts of these times when life was more predictable. Singing the songs and dancing the dances of that time makes these memories palpable.

When it is time for bed, playing music may be a calming influence. The best source for inducing sleep is very familiar and comforting music. Another candidate is music that has elements of the lullaby: simple, repetitive melodies, a rocking rhythm, consonant harmonies, and flowing phrases. But, for many, music attracts attention, and will interrupt the tired state that precedes sleep. In this case, music may be used to bring on a relaxed state of mind before attempting sleep. Winding down with music that gradually slows and reassures with pleasant memories may lull the listener into a dreamy condition that melts the insecurities experienced throughout the day.

48

I hope they know....gentle touch can give comfort and solace.

PATIENTS WITH MODERATE AND late stage Alzheimer's disease residing in long term care facilities rarely, if ever, receive 'nonprocedural touch', the touching that might be expected to promote comfort. They receive the touch that accompanies the handling that is associated with the activities of daily living or 'procedural' touch. Since touch for comfort or solace is not documented as part of a nursing care plan, like many of the special interactions between a doctor and his or her patient during the doctoring or practice of medicine, this kind of interaction falls into the region of "the art of nursing and medical care."

To know the moment when and how to hold someone with empathy and compassion as they cry or seem distressed is a learned skill, and few would deny the importance. With so many culturally diverse doctors, nurses and aides in our healthcare provider population today and with Alzheimer's patients that have severe cognitive impairment, there can be cultural confusion and even barriers to the nursing and doctoring tradition of comforting practices such as touch and comforting.

Touch itself may be considered tabu in many cultures and there is a strong concern for crossing cultural boundaries of either the person/patient, doctor or the nurse or aide. In the end, using ordered technical interventions such as medications for pain or tranquilizers for agitation and anxiety, specifically ordered by a physician and showing charted interventions and reactions and responses remain the standard expected of visible therapies. This is not necessarily the case in home care, where caregivers seem to become "part of the family" and comforting may even be expected.

Researchers began as early as 1975 exploring the use of gentle touch and massage techniques with geriatric patients. Although early studies were small with limited results, massage, therapeutic touch, and the calming physical presence began to emerge in the 1990s as viable alternatives in dementia care. Various forms of gentle touch, such as hand treatments, proved effective in decreasing problematic behaviors, particularly wandering, and resisting. A study of in-home use of slow-stroke massage to the upper body showed a reduction of the physical behaviors, such as pacing, resisting and wandering as well. Other studies have shown therapeutic touch can elicit a relaxation response, which helped agitation without medication as well.

Many assisted-living facilities, hospices and Day Programs have staff members and directors who are aware of the benefits of massage and bodywork for their residents and participants. Others still require help in recognizing the need. It only takes one episode where the family or caregivers of an Alzheimer's patient notice the positive response and benefit of gentle touch to show that the use of gentle touch and massage is as viable a part of a patient's care as nursing or social work, bathing or the feeding of a meal.

Quality of life and the dignity of human life are cemented in the bonds that coexist between human beings as they provide comfort and solace, and the sense of touch is integral to provide comfort.

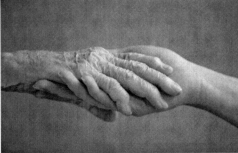

49

I hope they know....when to think about placement in a care facility.

THE GREATEST DETERMINING FACTORS in a family's decision to consider placement in a residential care facility are the behavioral and psychiatric symptoms. Consider too that there are many significant threats to the safety of the patient with progressive dementia in the home. Dementia can make day-to-day life more difficult. Little things like forgetting to turn the gas off or letting the bathwater overflow can cause great damage and may put the person with dementia and others in danger. Wandering out of the home onto a busy street or taking off in the car can also endanger others. Caregiver burnout is another factor that supports placement. Even though any one of a number of causes may necessitate placement, each family has their own threshold. Consider these examples. If the patient continues wandering and gets lost, interventions by local police and elder services may necessitate placement if the family cannot provide 24 hour monitoring or supervision at home, even if the dementia symptoms are only mild to moderate. Specialized feeding techniques to avoid choking may require thirty minutes or more at least three times a day to provide the nutrition and liquids needed. The daily need for assistance with getting in and out of bed, getting dressed and undressed, toileting, grooming and other activities during the day will all require assistance. If the caregiver is also elderly and frail, or ill, statistics show they will suffer a health decline in an attempt to provide care and may even need hospitalization.

There should be no shame or guilt associated with providing safety. Pushing to the extremes of tolerance may show devotion, but also rapidly expend the emotional and physical resources of the care giver. Heroics and denying oneself sleep, emotional support with friends and loved ones, or quiet private time are not necessary to prove or show your loyalty and devotion to a beloved family member if they are ill. Providing a safe environment is. Team work provides the best care. If this cannot be provided, placement is the solution for safety, optimal quality professional medical care and the best quality of life for the patient. The Appendix lists the various options for placement and long-term care alternatives.

50
I hope they know....life review with memorabilia can help cope.

LIFE REVIEW IS A precious gift of memories. Families can create an heirloom to be treasured by recording a written legacy using poetry. You and your family can create scrapbooks using photographs, collages, anything, even pieces of clothing and mementos once treasured by your loved one. Anything you chose can be put into a life review piece.

Looking back and sharing special memories can be both rewarding and entertaining, especially for an early dementia patient, but also for families of those with patients who no longer have family memories at all. Life review is designed to help a person tell his or her life story. Page by page, the life of the patient can be told, using stories of the family, adult life, childhood and extended family members. Such efforts can provide other family members with an emotional bond and connection to the patient through old experiences as well. It is also an heirloom that can be passed on to succeeding generations.

More recent research has proven that life review can improve an ill person's self-esteem, well-being and satisfaction with life. It can also be a project for family members of a patient with dementia to cope with their sense of grief and loss.

Experts offer the following tips for journaling and scrapbook making:
- Break the project into segments.
- Let photos or keepsakes trigger memories.
- Include as many details as possible, such as descriptions of smells, sights and sounds.
- Add names and dates.

- Don't worry about spelling and grammar.
- Let memories flow naturally.

Whether you follow these steps on your own or join a life review group, let your thoughts guide you through an insightful journey as you record a lasting legacy. There are also published guides to help you create a life review book if you need further guidance.

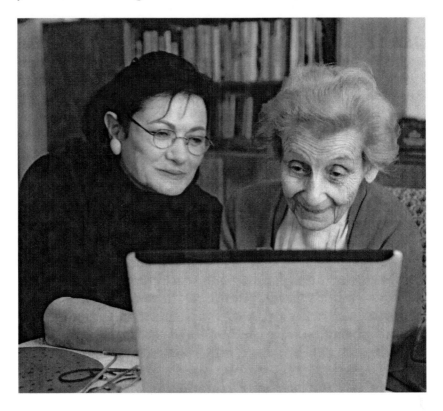

51
I hope they know....the grief and bereavement process is different.

DEMENTIA ILLNESSES GENERATE GRIEF and bereavement that is uncharacteristic of losses due to other forms of illness or death because they can occur over much longer periods. This ongoing process may be protracted over years as the illness progresses. Typically the most significant period of grief and bereavement starts in the period after death.

Grief is often expressed by feelings such as anger, guilt, sadness or loneliness. Grief affects us in other ways as well and can have an impact on our overall sense of wellbeing and general health.

Bereavement is the way we process grief. Each of us grieves in our own way, affected by such factors as our cultural norms, our gender and unique circumstances surrounding the loss. Every loss is unique. Losses are not only the end of life with death, also miscarriages, infertility, and loss of a lifetime job or position or a divorce can generate grief and bereavement as well.

Complicated grief is usually present when loss events are compounded, with multiple events occurring over a short period of time. This is often the case for elderly folks with other deaths of family and friends and other family changes. Perhaps the loss is a move from one home to another, often smaller home, necessitating upheaval and the loss of personal effects. Or even a bigger move to another city or state to be closer to younger family members, leaving behind support groups and friends.

Early on, the caregiver of a person with dementia may grieve the loss of freedom to work or to pursue other activities. The disease may cause the significant loss of finances or a lifestyle which was once enjoyed by both.

Later on, it is the loss in the ability to be recognized that is the hardest sense of loss to bear. It is the total loss of the person you once knew, the relationship you once enjoyed, their companionship, and special understanding and love between each other. It may feel as if a death has occurred, but physically, it has not. Although the relationship seems very nearly over, you are unable to mourn fully because the person is still alive. A sense of loss is one of the most powerful feelings that care givers experience. Often, loved ones of patients are shocked to find that they sometimes wish that the person were dead. This feeling alone can trigger powerful emotional conflicts and guilt. It may help to know that such feelings are normal and that other people experience similar reactions.

Dr. Elizabeth Kübler-Ross, a psychologist, contributed much to our understanding of grief and bereavement. In her studies in the 1970's, she outlined the various stages of these emotions.

- Stage 1- Shock and denial
- Stage 2- Anger
- Stage 3- Bargaining
- Stage 4- Depression
- Stage 5- Acceptance

It is best to acknowledge that grieving will be an up and down process no matter what the circumstances. In the earlier stages, you may swing between shock and wild optimism of a cure or improvement from new medications. At other times, you may feel overwhelmed by sadness or anger. Some people just feel numb. Later, when you have accepted the situation, you may find that there are periods when you can cope well. In other people, they find that they grieve so much during the course of the illness that they have no strong feelings left when the person with a dementia illness dies. Other people experience a range of overwhelming reactions at different times. These reactions can occur at any time after the diagnosis is made and include numbness, as though their feelings are frozen, inability to accept the situation, hysteria, and shock. These feeling occur even if death has been expected for a long time.

After the passing has occurred, caregivers and loved ones should be prepared for the fact that it may take them a long time to come to terms with the person's death, especially if the care giving was a full-time job. The passing will leave a void. The care giver may feel very unconfident at first and find it difficult to make decisions, make polite conversation or cope with social gatherings. They may feel very tired. It is best to take things slowly and make sure that there is plenty of support from family and friends, professionals and other former care givers in support groups or hospice programs or religious organizations. Accept that even though you may generally be coping, there will be times when you feel particularly sad or upset. Try to avoid making any major decisions in the early months if you are still feeling shocked and vulnerable.

There will come the time when you are ready to re-establish your own life and move forward. Events such as anniversaries, holiday seasons or birthdays may be distressing. If they are, ask friends and family for support. Stay in close touch with your own doctor. During these periods you may be likely to be more vulnerable to physical illness as well as to anxiety or depression. If after 6 months you are still not coping well, professional care may help. Seek the help of a bereavement specialist. They are understanding professionals with whom you can talk about your feelings to.

Don't bottle up your feelings. Don't repress your feelings and find a safe way to release them.

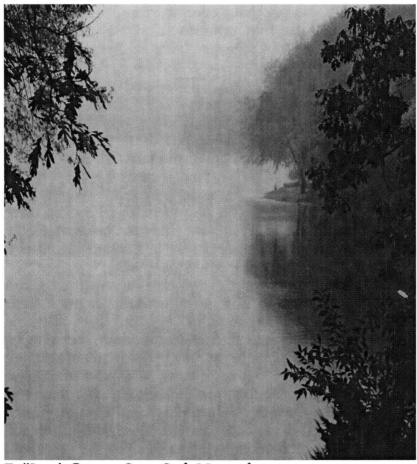

ZoëLewis©2007 Cape Cod, Massachusetts

Wind walker
He dances among the stars
and walks on the wind.
Death is a horizon.

Heavenward
Guided by the stars,
You journeyed beyond dream's edge,
In hushed reverence.

In God's Time
A blink of an eye
One thousand years in Heaven.
No separation.

Love Lives
Death came,
Taking him from our sight,
But not from our hearts.
Love lives on
Past the stilled night.

Debbi Dickinson© 2006

53

I hope they know....how to find and accept spiritual support.

ALL OF US FROM time to time search for answers to life's difficult questions. We don't need to be sick or dying to have existential concerns. We may ask ourselves about the existence of God or the injustice of suffering after reports of natural disasters where tens of thousands are killed in minutes, or ongoing bloodshed from wars that kill thousands of innocents. We may ponder why we still have starvation and depravation of water, or the senseless acts of teenage rampage killings. We may want to talk about life after death or make peace within our hearts when misery has us feeling down or overcome with grief. When we have witnessed personal tragedy with our own suffering we may feel unworthy of peace and salvation. We may not understand compassion for others. We may want to take care of unfinished business within our own souls to help us find that peace before we look outside of ourselves to help others.

Spiritual care and support are not necessarily religious. Its goal is to help a person achieve inner peace. No one philosophy or religious or spiritual belief has the answers to life's mysteries or holds any secrets. There is unity in all of the beliefs of one thing—that we are all and everything from one source and that the peace we are seeking outside of ourselves is actually within and has been and will be always.

Spiritual care can come solely from within you, without others presence. It can be guided with meditation, or reading books or hearing seminars on spiritual growth. Personal spiritual care is more difficult when you are in a state of crisis, but often that is when it seems to be needed most and the first steps are taken towards greater awareness. Spiritual care can also be a form of counseling that helps you find the answers to your questions. There is no requirement that you believe in a particular religion or that you believe in God. If you seek spiritual care, you will find help to tend to your own needs as a spiritual being. And it helps heal the pain you may feel about your life and what you're going through.

God has a name in every religion and the powers of God are omnipotent and universal in everyone. This is the lesson of most religions. Religious care is given in the context of the shared religious beliefs, values, liturgies and lifestyle of a faith community. Every one of us can make the personal choice to reach out to a religious organization. Most accept any follower.

Whether you choose spiritual care and support or religious support, studies have demonstrated spiritual well-being can offer a hope for peace in your heart and soul. Whether you pray, chant, or worship, your sense of peace comes from within, and there is no correct path or map for the fast road to heaven, bliss, nirvana or oneness.

Ask your local Alzheimer's Association or doctor for information about spiritual care for persons with dementia and for their caregivers. Private therapists in your community may offer spiritual counseling as well.

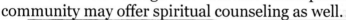

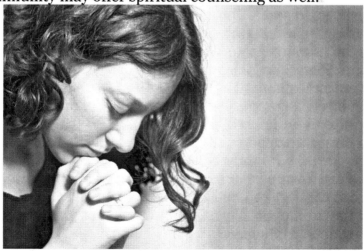

54
I hope they know....how to gain strength from caregiver support groups.

MANY CAREGIVERS STRUGGLE WITH feelings of guilt and anger, and need support and reassurance to remember that the disease is creating the intolerable behavior in their loved one, not the person they once knew. Previous poor habits can seem magnified though and intentional. Often, this can set off the old anger and frustration buttons that existed before the disease was diagnosed. These toxic feelings create resentment and will increase caregiver stress and are not helpful. They challenge your emotional intelligence even when you are aware of what is going on. Our emotional intelligence can be greatly tested with a loved one with Alzheimer's disease, but in the end, awareness can illuminate most problems.

Social support is important for caregivers whose own mental and physical health can be negatively affected by the emotional burden and sadness of caring for someone with Alzheimer's disease. There are a number of sources of help, including organizations, newsletters, books, and computer sites on the Internet. The top Internet and Alzheimer's Organizations and Aging Services are listed in this book. If you are not a computer user, then get personalized help with outreach groups. You can use the telephone to connect to groups to get printed information.

Joining a support group allows caregivers to meet and share ideas with others who are coping with similar problems. Group members will have similar experiences and can comfort you and often have good ideas for dealing with day-to-day problems. Many have been there and are willing to help others.

You can locate the nearest support group by contacting the Alzheimer's Association or sometimes community organizations such as a senior center or your local hospital or a hospice program, if hospice services are already in place.

Sometimes a private therapist can be helpful in dealing with stress, anxiety, or depression in family caregivers. There should be no shame in needing help with feelings of conflict, anger or guilt. It happens to many people and counseling can help with these feelings. Religious organizations and spiritual support groups can also help.

Sometimes caregivers find it very difficult to arrange time to attend meetings, appointments or groups outside the home. In this case, you might consider one of the toll-free telephone help lines. Trained peer counselors are available to answer questions or just talk about problems you may be having 24 hours a day, 7 days a week. You never need to feel alone. With so many people with this disease, new services are being created and new organizations founded ready to help.

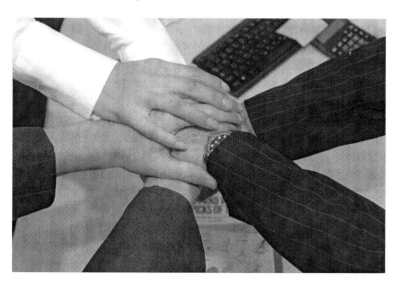

55

I hope they know....palliative medical treatments and care are options.

PALLIATIVE CARE IS A choice of medical care that has as primary goals pain management for suffering and medical treatments that improve the quality of life, without attempting to prolong or hasten death. The palliative care approach attempts to eliminate or control symptoms and provide care and comfort in the late and final stages of the disease. The specialized team approach results in increased patient and family satisfaction and compliance. When these programs are located in hospitals, it awards the facility the highest care and quality standard rankings for end-of-life care. Check with your local hospitals and see if they offer palliative care experts or a consultation service.

Palliative care programs are now in hundreds of hospitals in the USA and thousands of hospitals worldwide. Patients electing these services are those with any life-threatening illness, including moderate and late stage dementia and Alzheimer's disease. The care is offered in an interdisciplinary team approach and offered in conjunction with all other appropriate forms of medical treatment. In particular, for patients with advanced illness due to Alzheimer's disease and other forms of dementia, palliative care programs structure a variety of hospital and long-term care facility resources to effectively deliver the highest quality of care to these patients. The team approach includes medical and nursing specialists, social workers, clergy, and others. Vigorous pain and symptom control is integrated into all stages of treatment. Successful palliative care programs have used an array of delivery systems from consultative services to inpatient units.

Hospice and Palliative Medicine is now recognized as a medical subspecialty by the American Board of Internal Medicine and the American Board of Hospice and Palliative Medicine. Fellowship training will now be required and a board certification examination taken for members to become board certified practitioners. Nurses as well can take advanced degree training in this developing field of medical care. The mission of the American Board of Hospice and Palliative Medicine is to promote excellence in the delivery of medical care to all patients with advanced, progressive illness through the development of standards for training and practice in palliative medicine.

The Center to Advance Palliative Care (CAPC) provides health care professionals with the tools, training and technical assistance necessary to start and sustain successful palliative care programs in hospitals and other health care settings. CAPC is a national organization dedicated to increasing the availability of quality palliative care services for people facing serious illness. Direction and technical assistance are provided by Mount Sinai School of Medicine. www.capc.org

The website is meant for professionals but it also offers a listing of the national hospital palliative care programs available today.

56
Surviving By Fanny Barry

AS A CANCER SURVIVOR, I celebrate life with a desire and need to improve the lives of others. Care from others, help, love and a deeper understanding of impermanence, have heightened my empathy, tolerance, laughter and understanding. I have found myself again and I am in a place where I need to give more to others than ever before. To survive, I have accepted so much from others, some very close and some very new acquaintances brought me through the disease. No one makes the survivor journey alone.

At first, I kept my "survivorship" fairly secret. Probably the same way a diagnosis of Alzheimer's might be kept secret. I don't tell everyone. It frightens some and makes some people uneasy. It is about death, I know. A lot of people don't want to hear it, don't want to think about it. I understand that. Sometimes I don't want to think about it either. So I try not to talk too much about it. But it is there. And, more and more, as I become comfortable with the fact, with the term "survivor", I share.

Each time I share I tell myself "ok" first. There is this little voice inside me that whispers "Go ahead. They, he, she, might want to know. It is ok. Say it. It is not a bad thing." So I say it. Selectively, more and more. And people do want to know. Often they share their stories. So many have been touched. "My mother died of the disease." "My sister had it and is doing well." "My friend was just diagnosed." "I am a survivor too." Somehow it gives people permission to share their stories. Somehow it takes away my embarrassment of the diagnosis and gives me pride in my survivorship. Too, it frees those with whom I share. By sharing my survivorship, I enable the little voice inside of them to whisper "go ahead, she wants to know. It is ok." It enables them to be heard, to not be embarrassed. And so we share. Often, there is a bond. Always, there is comfort. Realistically, it is how I survived. I told others I had cancer and they helped me. Now as I tell people and we share our stories, there is the realization of a problem. We realize there is a need to solve it or at least to help each other try.

Communicating the existence of the disease is a first step to enabling people to help each other. It is how we stop denying that we could have the disease. It is how we start accepting that we need to do something. That is why I started my non-profit. That is why I wrote my books. That is why I tell people, "I am a survivor." When we share the knowledge, we are able to help each other. When we share the knowledge, we diminish the shame, the doubt, the fear.

Those touched by breast cancer and I believe most who have faced death, either themselves or through a loved one are changed by the experience. "Of course" you say. Every experience changes us, adds to the fabric of our being. But my experience surviving breast cancer has changed me in ways I would never have imagined. It has changed my family and friends, probably in ways they could never imagine. It showed me, and them, my strengths and my weaknesses. It took me to the edge and back. I know it took people I love and who love me to the edge and back. We are all survivors. But it also developed in me and in them a greater sense of empathy, tolerance and a greater need to share our lives with others as fortunate as we are— fortunate to be alive and to live every day. Fortunate to breathe each breath in awareness of the gift of life and in the awareness that we need to help each other do the same.

Communication can be a key to survivorship. Communication can be a key to those who may not survive so that they may have a better quality of life during their illness. It enables those who love them to come back from the edge. There is a parallel in all life death situations. Alzheimer's disease is no different. There is an embarrassment I am sure. But there also needs to be that little voice inside that can speak up to share, selectively.

That little voice that says, "It is ok, go ahead, they, he, she might want to know. It is ok. Say it. It is not a bad thing."

Sharing our situations, our experiences, our needs will engender a commonality of compassion, a desire to improve each persons experience with disease, with life and death situations and will allow survivors and support systems to give back in some way, because no one survives alone. And for those who leave, no one leaves any one behind. We all touch each other and we leave a void when we go where others cannot follow. That void can be filled with empathy, compassion, an ability to help and give to others and a community of care.

57
I hope they know....hospice programs can be a resource.

THE FIRST HOSPICE IN the United States was established in New Haven, Connecticut in 1974 but it was during the 1960's, that Dr. Cicely Saunders, a British physician began the modern hospice movement by establishing St. Christopher's Hospice near London. Today there are more than 3,200 hospice programs in the United States, Puerto Rico and Guam.

Many people are still unaware that hospice care is a covered benefit under Medicare but is strictly for patients with a prognosis of 6 months or less. A patient can remain in hospice care beyond six months if a physician re-certifies that the patient is terminally ill. In other words, their prognosis is unchanged and they will likely succumb to their disease in 6 months or less.

There are many regulations and criteria for the hospice benefit, and in particular end-stage dementia has specific criteria for admission. Many physicians use the Global Deterioration Scale, listed in the appendix. Patients are generally eligible for service once they have reached stage 7, with very severe decline, weight loss, incontinence and immobility. While patients must have a doctor's referral to enter hospice, the patient, family and friends can initiate the process by contacting a local hospice program. This benefit covers all services, medications and equipment related to the illness. For example, physician services, nursing services, home health aides, medical equipment and supplies, counseling, trained volunteers, and bereavement services are inclusive in the hospice benefit. It does not cover the "room and board" expense of long-term care.

Keep in mind that hospice is not a place but a concept of care. Most hospice care is provided in the patient's home or family member's home. Usually end-stage dementia patients are cared for in nursing homes or long term care facilities at the end of their disease, and by then, many of the families have exhausted their resources and the patients "room" expense is fully covered by Medicaid. Inpatient hospice facilities are sometimes available to assist with care giving if the patient is cared for at home and the family requests respite care. This is medical care that is arranged with an inpatient hospice unit or skilled nursing facility for a short duration and is typically less than seven days. Respite care is covered by the hospice benefit.

Before providing care, the hospice staff meets with the patient, the patient's family and physicians and a hospice physician to discuss patient history, current physical symptoms and life expectancy. A plan of care is developed for the patient. This plan is regularly reviewed and revised according to the patient condition at team meetings that occur routinely with the entire team present, excluding the volunteers, but with the presence of the volunteer coordinator. These team meetings cover everything that has occurred regarding patient care issues yet the team manages changes and needs as they occur daily.

The Hospice Foundation of America has in depth hospice program information and a directory of hospice programs in your area. 800.854.3402
http://www.hospicefoundation.org

58
Forever Changing

YOUR SADNESS
Reminds me of autumn leaves.
Colors change, like youth,
Spectacular,
in their bleeding, fleeting efforts,
To remain green and attached
They fall to the ground,
Brown,
Crumpled,
And so we are forever changing.

Zoë Lewis, ©1999

59
Maintaining Balance by Kino MacGregor

My experience with Yoga and spiritual strength

CHALLENGING SITUATIONS OFTEN ARRIVE at the least convenient times. You get sick right the middle of a stressful period of your life. Or perhaps your dad is diagnosed with Alzheimer's right when you realize how much you love and miss him. You loose your job right when you need a promotion. You can't find a taxi when it's raining.

You create your reality by the thoughts that you think. Your attention is itself responsible for your life experience. No matter how awful the traffic jam is, how inconsiderate people may seem, or how sick your family members are, you are the one who is in control of your perception of reality.

Yet rather than collapse under the weight of the hardship, you can find your greatest spiritual strength in the midst of the roughest times. Regardless of what type of experience finds its way into your life, you always have power over your reaction to reality. In doing so, you are the true master of your own fate. Think that life is awful and it is...for you. Think that people are careless, blind and ignorant and they will be...to you. The power of positive thinking is a common topic of conversation, books and seminars in our post-new age, twenty-first century world. Most of us agree that it's a good idea to concentrate our thoughts towards a positive goal, rather than lull around in the doldrums of complaint and whine. The real question lies not in the debate about whether we can create our own reality or not, but rather in the how. I have dedicated my life in the yoga tradition. Yoga can be for anyone and benefits everyone who practices. Yoga may not be for you, but if you are interested to read about it, here it is in a nutshell.

Enter the five thousand year old tradition of which you take part when you practice yoga. Yoga is a true science of the mind where you actively practice choosing a peaceful response to distressful situations, thus giving you the tools for creating your reality in each moment. When you practice yoga, you watch your mind's reaction to touching the borders of your physical reality. Your inner dialogue in postures that seem impossible to you parallels your reaction to life situations that push the boundary of your "comfortability". Pushing these limits brings up fear, anger, sadness, frustration, and numerous other insidious emotions. It is easy to let your mind spin away into these temptations; however, with regular practice you will have the strength to remain calm, focused and aware. As you remain calm, you are able to choose a peaceful response to your experience and thereby create your own reality.

You can only start where you are, in the center of your created life experience and begin the dedicated, devotional path towards creating a peaceful life in the present moment, one step like one breath at a time. Yoga gives you the strength and spiritual willpower to face challenging situations when they arise in your life. Confrontation with some of the most difficult moments of your life tests what you've learned along the spiritual path. Diagnosed illness is perhaps one of the hardest things to face. Should you fight your way out of a defeatist victim-mentality? Or should you take a few breathes to ventilate your hostility and anger over the unfairness of the diagnosis of an incurable disease. Anger, whether my own or someone else's, has always been challenging for me. No matter how awful the situation, how righteous you are, how indignant or cynical you become, no matter how grand and tragic the loss, whatever emotions you feel, they are always your responsibility. You always have a choice about how you respond to life. You always have the power to choose a gracious way in and out of any situation. You are more powerful than any of life's fortunes or misfortunes.

The basic teaching of spiritual practice is to find yourself in the midst of your greatest challenge and stay. There is magic in staying with what Tibetan teacher Pema Chodron calls "the places that scare you". For in those truly empowering moments you bear witness to the law of impermanence. Whatever arises in your experience, no matter how solid and sticky, it too will change. All emotions flow if we don't hold onto them. Sooner or later, the seemingly solid righteousness of anger yields and gives way to the soft, forgiveness of peace and understanding. The greatest storm will pass and the sun will rise again another day. Albert Einstein says that you cannot solve a problem from the same level of thinking that created it. And so it is. Anger cannot create peace. The powerful choice to stay gives you the opportunity to create the space of transformation in your life today.

Every time you choose to respond peacefully to a difficult life situation, you practice the kind of spiritual strength it takes to maintain your equanimity in the face of the vicissitudes of life. It is easy to write and read about these things and harder yet to live them.

If you feel drawn to the deep inner work of yoga and spirituality, begin it now. Who you are matters to everyone in your life, especially to your loved ones, your self realization matters on so many levels. There is a world of deep connection and joy available to you right now. It starts with your experience and never ends. It is infinite. Just like you. Just like our connections.

60
I hope they know....a few of the dedicated Alzheimer's Organizations

- The National Institute on Aging
  www.nia.nih.gov

- Alzheimer's Disease Education and Referral Center
  (800) 438-4380
  www.nia.nih.gov/alzheimers

- The Alzheimer's Association National Chapter
  (800) 272-3900
  www.alz.org

- The Alzheimer's Research Foundation
  (877)4270220
  www.alzheimers-research.org

- The National Alzheimer's Coordination Center
  Internet Database
  www.alz.washington.edu

- The Alzheimer's Foundation of America
  (866)232-8484
  www.alzfdn.org

- Fischer Center for Alzheimer's Research
  Foundation
  (800) ALZINFO
  www.alzinfo.org

- www.ClinicalTrials.gov

Provides information about federally and privately supported clinical research in human volunteers

INTERNATIONAL ORGANIZATIONS

- Alzheimer's Society United Kingdom
  www.alzheimers.org.uk

- Alzheimer's Disease International (ADI)
  www.alz.co.uk

61
I hope they know....Aging Services Web Links

American Association of Retired Persons (AARP)
http://www.aarp.org
Administration on Aging (AOA)
http://www.aoa.gov
American Society on Aging
http://www.asaging.org/index.cfm
NADSA Directory of Adult Day Service Centers
http://www.nadsa.org
National Hospice and Palliative Care Organization
http://www.nhpco.org
National Institute on Aging
http://www.nia.nih.gov
Senior Job Bank
http://www.seniorjobbank.com
Robert Wood Johnson Foundation
http://www.rwjf.org
American Association of Homes and Services for the Aging (AAHSA)
http://www.aahsa.org/
National PACE Organization
http://www.npaonline.org
National Council on the Aging, Inc.
http://www.ncoa.org
SPRY Foundation
http://www.spry.org
National Association of Area Agencies on Aging
http://www.n4a.org
Department of Health and Human Services Eldercare
http://www.eldercare.gov/Eldercare/Public/Home.asp

62
Contributing Authors Biographies

Elizabeth Cockey, M.A.T is a Baltimore based art therapist and consultant to healthcare facilities about the utilization of art programs for recovery. Elizabeth has worked with Alzheimer's and stroke dementia clients for the past 15 years. She holds degrees in art, psychology, and a master's degree in art therapy. Elizabeth is also an artist, a motivational speaker and the author of *Drawn from Memory: A Personal Story of Healing through Art*. She is a member of the American Art Therapy Association and the American Society on Aging. htpp://www.elizabethcockey.com

Suzanne B. Hanser, EdD, MT-BC is Chair of the Music Therapy Department at Berklee College of Music, Boston, Massachusetts. She is Past President of the World Federation Music Therapy Association and the American Music Therapy Association. She is currently a Research Associate and Music Therapist at the Dana-Farber Cancer Institute in Boston. She has more than 200 scientific publications and three published books including *The New Music Therapist's Handbook*, in its third edition and *When You Wish upon a Star*. She is an internationally recognized speaker at psychiatry, psychology, education, music, gerontology and special education conferences.

Her past academic responsibilities are numerous and include positions as the former professor and chair of music therapy at the University of the Pacific, and past program director of the Alzheimer's Association greater San Francisco Bay area. She has received numerous research grants and a National Service Award from the National Institute on Aging. Her work has been covered on local and national television programs and other forms of media coverage.

"These days there's a lot of attention to New Age philosophies and approaches to life, and drumming circles have become very popular. People get a lot out of that, and for some it's a spiritual experience. They think that's music therapy. But music therapy is scientific in addition to being an artistic endeavor. It's really a structured and formulaic approach to meeting individual needs. Music therapy is the systematic approach to using music to meet the specific need of a person or group. Music has to come so naturally to the therapist that he or she can be totally with the client and tuned in to what he or she needs at the moment, totally empathizing and understanding not only what the person's saying, but what they're feeling."
http://www. Berklee.edu/faculty

Myron Weiner, M.D. is a geriatric psychiatrist whose primary interest is in managing the emotional and behavioral symptoms of dementing illness. Dr. Weiner is Professor of Psychiatry and Neurology at UT Southwestern Medical Center at Dallas, Texas, where he formerly headed the Geriatric Psychiatry Residency Program and Clinical Core of the UT Southwestern Alzheimer's Disease Center. He holds the Aradine S. Ard Chair in Brain Science and the Dorothy L. and John P. Harbin Chair in Alzheimer's Disease Research. He has more than 200 scientific publications to his credit, including the third edition of *The Dementias: Diagnosis, Treatment, and Research*, published by American Psychiatric Publishing, Inc. in 2003. He is senior editor of the American Psychiatric Publishing, *Textbook of Alzheimer Disease and Other Dementias,* which will appear in the fall of 2008.

His primary research is in treatment of Alzheimer's disease and its behavioral/psychological consequences, including impact on caregivers. His exploration of the impact of cardiovascular risk factors in the development of Alzheimer's disease in American Indians led him to establish a telemedicine link for dementia evaluation and follow up with the Choctaw Nation of Oklahoma.

Dr. Weiner has received the Texas Society of Psychiatric Physicians Psychiatric Excellence Award, is a Distinguished Life Fellow of the American Psychiatric Association, and holds the Castle Connolly Medical Ltd. Award for America's Top Doctors.

Dr. Weiner and colleagues developed the Quality of Life in Late-stage Alzheimer's Disease (QUALID) scale, now used around the world in studies of interventions for late-stage Alzheimer disease patients. He also was a developer of the Test of Everyday Functional Abilities (TEFA), an ecologically valid scale for use in determining level of competence at activities of daily living. http://www.utsouthwestern.edu

Patricia Munhall, EdD, NCPsyA, CHt, ARNP, has twenty-three years practicing psychoanalysis and psychodynamic psychotherapy. She is the founder and director of the International Institute of Human Understanding. Her special clinical interests span a wide range of clients and she has facilitated quality of life and emotional growth and personality integration for a diverse client population in addition to many other areas of interest and clinical specialization.

She has been a former Professor of Nursing for thirty years at various universities, including Hunter College, CUNY, Teachers College and Columbia University.

Dr. Munhall has authored 11 books and over 60 articles. She writes of the experiential nature of man, woman and family in the 21st century. *The Emergence of Man into the 21st Century, The Emergence of the Family Into the 21st Century, The Emergence of Women Into the 21st Century, Research: A Qualitative Perspective* (3rd edition), *Qualitative Research Reports and Proposals: A Guide, Revisioning Phenomenology: Nursing & Health Science Research, In Women's Experience (Volume I), In Women's Experience Volume II.*

Dr. Munhall is a recognized international speaker on numerous topics including ethics, the art of listening, family dynamics and depression.

This year she was voted "Best Of" Psychotherapists by *Family, Health, and Fitness* magazine. She is in clinical practice in Miami, Florida. http://www.iihu.org

Kino MacGregor, M.A. is the founder of Miami Life Center, an urban retreat space dedicated to the study of yoga, holistic health and consciousness. Located in Miami Beach, Florida, the Miami Life Center offers daily yoga classes, life coaching, and trainings as well as workshops with international leaders in yoga and spirituality. Kino is a Ph.D. student in holistic health with a Master's Degree in holistic health from New York University.

Kino and the Miami Life Center have been featured in *Yoga Journal, Yoga Magazine, Yoga Joyful Living, the Miami Herald, EuroMan, Travel & Leisure Magazine, Ocean Drive Magazine, Daily Candy, Six Degrees Magazine,* as well as appearing on *The CBS Today Show.* Kino is one of a select few people to receive the certification to teach Ashtanga Yoga by its founder Sri K. Pattabhi Jois in Mysore, India. Perhaps the youngest woman to hold this title, she has completed the challenging Third Series and is now learning the Fourth Series. Traveling internationally, she leads classes, privates, workshops and retreats in traditional Ashtanga yoga, holistic health and total life transformation. http://www.miamilifecenter.com

Fanny Barry, M.S. is a writer, artist, and breast cancer survivor. She has a Master of Science in Communications and Public Relations, and a Bachelor of Science in General Engineering, both from Boston University. A native of Boston, Massachusetts, she completed treatment for breast cancer in 2004. During her treatment and into recuperation she kept journals of her experience which became the basis for her illustrated book series: *I Wish I Knew; I Wish I Knew How to Help,* and *I Wish I Knew Who*

I Have Become. These books represent her personal observations on how her life and the lives of those closest to her changed while undergoing treatment for cancer. Cancer left her with a great desire to share her insights with other patients and survivors to help them cope emotionally. After recuperating, she developed That Barry Girl Foundation, Thriving, not just Surviving to accomplish this desire: to offer emotional, financial and recuperative support for breast cancer patients and survivors. http://www.thatbarrygirl.org

Debbi Dickinson, B.A. has a B.A. degree in Psychology from Westfield State College, Westfield, Massachusetts. She holds numerous advanced certifications and completed the Bereavement Specialist Skills Training and Certification Program by the American Hospice Foundation and World Pastoral Care Center. Debbi's work has appeared in over 400 publications. She is the author of *HeartSongs* and *Whispers in the Wind.* Debbi gives presentations nationwide to the bereaved as well as to professionals. www.debbidickinson.com

Appendix

1. The Global Deterioration Scale for Dementing Illnesses

Some health-care professionals use the Global Deterioration Scale, also called the Reisberg Scale, to measure progression of Alzheimer's disease. This scale divides Alzheimer's disease into seven stages of decreasing ability.

Stage 1: No cognitive decline
- Experiences no problems in daily living.

Stage 2: Very mild cognitive decline
- Forgets names and locations of objects.
- May have trouble finding words.

Stage 3: Mild cognitive decline
- Has difficulty traveling to new locations.
- Has difficulty handling problems at work.

Stage 4: Moderate cognitive decline
- Has difficulty with complex tasks (finances, shopping, planning dinner for guests).

Stage 5: Moderately severe cognitive decline
- Needs help to choose clothing.
- Needs prompting to bathe.

Stage 6: Severe cognitive decline
- Needs help putting on clothing.
- Requires assistance bathing; may have a fear of bathing.
- Has decreased ability to use the toilet or is incontinent

Stage 7: Very severe cognitive decline
- Vocabulary becomes limited, eventually declining to single words.
- Loses ability to walk and sit.
- Becomes unable to smile.

Modified from Global Deterioration Scale, Reisberg, 1982. Reisberg, B., Ferris, S.H., de Leon, M.J., and Crook, T., *American Journal of Psychiatry*, 139:1136-1139, 1982.

2. The Three Stages of Dementia Illness Scale

Early stage

A person in this stage will usually be aware of the diagnosis and will be able to participate in decisions affecting future care. Symptoms can include mild forgetfulness and communication difficulties, such as finding the right word and following a conversation. Some people stay involved in activities while others become passive or withdrawn. The individual may also be frustrated by changing abilities and may become depressed or anxious. It is important to monitor the emotional well-being of the person. This stage is when they may still drive.

Abilities Affected	Typical Symptoms
Mental Abilities	• mild forgetfulness • difficulty learning new things and following conversations • difficulty concentrating or limited attention span • problems with orientation, such as getting lost or not following directions • communication difficulties such as finding the right word
Moods and Emotions	• mood shifts • depression
Behaviors	• passiveness • withdrawal from usual activities • restlessness
Physical Abilities	• mild co-ordination problems

Middle stage

This stage brings a further decline in the person's mental and physical abilities. Memory will continue to deteriorate as the person forgets personal history and no longer recognizes family and friends. Increased confusion and disorientation to time and place will result in requiring assistance in many daily tasks, such as dressing, bathing, using the toilet.

In this stage, some people become restless and pace or wander. In response to the loss of abilities, a person may react in a number of ways. For example, he or she may become less involved in activities or repeat the same action or word over and over again. It can be helpful to understand more about the disease and begin to develop strategies to deal with these situations in this stage.

Abilities Affected	Typical Symptoms
Mental Abilities	• continued memory problems • forgetfulness about personal history • inability to recognize friends and family • disorientation about time and place
Moods and Emotions	• personality change • confusion • anxiety/apprehension • suspiciousness • mood shifts • anger • sadness/depression • hostility
Behaviors	• declining ability to concentrate • restlessness (pacing, wandering) • repetition • delusions • aggression • uninhibited behavior • passiveness
Physical Abilities	• assistance required for daily tasks (e.g., dressing, bathing, using the toilet) • disrupted sleep patterns • appetite fluctuations • language difficulties • visual spatial problems

Late stage

In this last stage, the person becomes unable to remember, communicate or look after them self. Care is required 24 hours a day. Eventually, the person will become bed-ridden, have difficulty eating or swallowing, and lose control of bodily functions. This stage eventually ends with the person's death, often from secondary complications such as pneumonia or other infections.

Abilities Affected	Typical Symptoms
Mental Abilities	• loss of ability to remember, communicate or function • inability to process information • severe speaking difficulties • severe disorientation about time, place and people
Moods and Emotions	• possible withdrawal
Behaviors	• non-verbal methods of communicating (eye contact, crying, groaning)
Physical Abilities	• sleeps longer and more often • becomes immobile (bed-ridden) • loses ability to speak • loses control of bladder and bowels • has difficulty eating and/or swallowing • unable to dress or bathe • may lose weight

3. Driving Safely Checklist- 30 High Risk Warning Signs

The driving behaviors listed below could cause safety problems. **They are ranked from minor to serious.** Here's how to use this list:

• Observe driving over time, keeping notes to help you understand **changes** in driving ability.

• Look for a **pattern** of warning signs and for an increase in the frequency of occurrence.

1. Decrease in confidence while driving
2. Difficulty turning to see when backing up
3. Riding the brake
4. Easily distracted while driving
5. Other drivers often honk horns
6. Incorrect signaling
7. Parking inappropriately
8. Hitting curbs
9. Scrapes or dents on the car, mailbox or garage
10. Increased agitation or irritation when driving
11. Failure to notice important activity on the side of the road
12. Failure to notice traffic signs
13. Trouble navigating turns
14. Driving at inappropriate speeds
15. Not anticipating potential dangerous situations
16. Cannot manage unless another passenger is a copilot
17. Bad judgment on making left hand turns
18. Near misses
19. Delayed response to unexpected situations
20. Moving into wrong lane
21. Running out of gas frequently
22. Confusion at exits
23. Ticketed moving violations or warnings
24. No current registration or driver's license
25. Getting lost in familiar places
26. Difficulty maintaining lane position
27. Confusing the gas and brake pedals
28. Failure to stop at stop sign or red light

29. Stopping in traffic for no apparent reason
30. Car accident

4. Long-term Care Placement Alternatives

Skilled Nursing

Skilled nursing facilities are licensed to provide 24-hour medical services by registered nurses and other professionals for the chronically ill not requiring hospitalization. This is the highest level of nursing care available outside of hospitalization. There are many restrictions and medical insurance regulations. Your doctor will need to be involved with arrangements for this kind of care. You cannot "elect" to have skilled nursing care it must be indicated by a skilled *nursing* need for ongoing nursing care. The need must be other than assistance with an activity of daily living.

Alzheimer's Assisted Living

Alzheimer's assisted living provides 24-hour assistance with dressing, bathing, meals, medication monitoring, and transfer assistance. These large and small facilities have secure areas both inside and outside where residents are free to move about. Private fee and some insurance with long term care provisions.

Alzheimer's Skilled Nursing

Alzheimer's skilled nursing provides long-term, 24-hour nursing care. This is the highest level of nursing care available outside of hospitalization. Some facilities accept only "non-wandering" Alzheimer's patients. Accept private fee and some insurance with long term care provisions.

Care Alternatives to Senior Housing
Adult Day Care Programs

Adult day care programs are for seniors needing a place to stay during the day because they have dementia or physical limitations and cannot be left alone. These programs provide purpose and stimulation through planned activities. Accept fee for service and PACE, Medicaid.

Homemakers and Companions

Homemakers and companions provide in-home support services on a daily or weekly basis to individuals not in need of medical assistance. These services can include housekeeping, errands, respite care, meal preparation, and social contact. Accept fee for service, Medicare and Medicaid, insurance.

Hospices

Hospices provide individuals facing terminal illness with care at home or in a healthcare facility. The goal is to assist patients to live the last stage of their lives with dignity. Most hospices will accept Medicare, Medicaid, insurance, and private pay. Room and board not a covered expense.

5. Test to Assess Caregiver Burnout

Self-administered survey completed by caregiver
Categories A-D determine variables of burnout

Answers rated as 0-never to 4-nearly always)

A. General feelings
   1. Not enough time for self
   2. Over-taxed with responsibilities
   3. Lost control of life
B. Feelings regarding caring for relative
   1. Uncertain about what to do for relative
   2. Feeling that should do more for relative
   3. Feeling that could do a better job of caring
   4. Overall level of burden
C. Sense of responsibility
   1. Excessive help requests
   2. Level of need that impaired relative depends on caregiver
   3. Sense that all responsibility falls on one caregiver
   4. Fear of future regarding impaired relative
   5. Fear of not enough money to care for relative
   6. Fear of not able to continue caring for relative
   7. Wish to leave care of relative to someone else
D. Feelings when together with impaired relative
   1. Sense of strain
   2. Anger
   3. Embarrassed
   4. Uncomfortable about having friends over

5.   Relationship with relative negatively impacts social life
6.   Impacts other relationships with family and friends
7.   Impacts caregiver health
8.   Privacy

Interpretation:

No or minimal burden: 0 to 20

Mild to moderate burden: 21 to 40

Moderate to severe burden: 41 to 60

Severe burden: 61 to 88

Modified from the study by Kumamoto, Keigo, Masakazu,Washio, and Arai Yumiko in <u>Geriatrics & Gerontology International,</u> S1 (2004), "Assessment of family caregiver burden in the context of the LTC insurance system."

6. Art Therapy Projects and Suggestions By Elizabeth Cockey

- Keep it simple. Painting and sculpting are activities most individuals with mild to moderate dementia can accomplish. It is reasonable to give free rein. Otherwise, you can provide some guidance. The purpose is to interact.

-

- Evoke memories. Suggest drawing a farm, a snowman or other images that are familiar or can evoke childhood memories. Get out the family photo album and "remember" who's who in the photographs. Look for simple things to draw in the photos like a flower or tree, a table. Simple paper and colored pencils or markers are appropriate for everyone, but watercolors and nontoxic paints can be purchased in drugstores and supermarkets.

- Play it safe with the materials you choose. At one art therapy group, several individuals tried to use the paintbrushes like silverware; others attempted to drink the non-toxic paint that had been squirted into cups. The best way to ensure safety is to use materials that would be harmless if swallowed. Check all labels and only purchase paint and other materials that are non-toxic. Just in case: homemade clay and paint are preferable to store-bought versions because they can be made with ingredients that are edible. I have included the recipes.

- Select stimulating materials. Individuals in mid-to-late stage dementia often respond best to brightly colored paints and organic materials such as homemade clay. Other objects like cardboard candy boxes, empty cigar boxes, balls of yarn, old photograph albums, and pieces of cotton material also are favored. Glue or paste needs to be non-toxic.

- Taking the time to create a work area initially will be beneficial in that it provides habitual orientation; the key to recapturing a distracted or confused mind. I would suggest setting up an old card table to do the art projects, but the kitchen table will do just fine. I store all of my miscellaneous materials in a cardboard box. Having all the materials in one box makes it easier to stash away under the kitchen sink or in a closet. Lighting is also important. Have the work area situated in front of a window or use a table lamp. Low light is troublesome for anyone who can't see well.

- Create a comfortable setting. Play music in the background—soothing but not distracting. Provide lighting that is adequate, but not too bright. Ideally, art therapy works best after an individual has eaten breakfast and gotten dressed in the morning. Interactive programs in the late afternoon are not as effective because many individuals in the middle to late stages of dementia are tired or thinking about eating dinner and can be easily distracted.

- Give sensible, basic and concise directions before you begin any project. Remember "over there" means very little to a person who is visually impaired. Give specific directions with regard to right or left, between, behind, next to and the like. Be aware that your sense of touch may not be like that of your grandmother. Asking "Can you feel that?" is not always the best thing to say. Some textures bother people so be aware how the paints feels if it gets on his or her hands. I have found that many older adults don't like getting their hands dirty. Use disposable latex gloves that can be purchased in drug stores for projects that involve sculpting or mixing.

- Avoid long lulls in the activity when nothing is taking place. In-other-words, when you are doing any art project it's not the best time to talk on the phone; even for a minute or two. I have had dementia patients drink the paint in a matter of seconds when my back was turned for "just a minute." Stand behind the person when you are showing them how to do something. I prefer to lean around someone and wrap my hands around their hands to demonstrate how to hold a paintbrush, or use scissors.

- Be positive! Aim for no-failure activities. Like all other adults, individuals, even mid-stage Alzheimer's patients want the painting to "look right", and they will become very critical of their work. You must continually reinforce the notion that they can become "real artists" one brushstroke at a time.

- Sustain focus. In addition to being positive reinforcements and compliments such as "terrific" and "great job" can help keep someone focused. It is also easy to draw individuals in by asking personal questions. For example, try, "What do you think your daughter is going to say when she sees this painting?"

- Talk about the artwork. If your client or parent is still verbal, ask about the artwork or a favorite color. Open-ended questions will tap into memories, spark conversations and encourage socialization. Use your knowledge about the individual, such as past hobbies, former professions and family life. A drawing of sunflowers could lead to a discussion about gardening with someone who had enjoyed that hobby in the past, for instance.

7. Homemade Sculpting Clay and Paint Recipes

Sculpting Clay

This clay is simple and easy to make. Many probably have the ingredients lying around the kitchen—but it not they are readily available in any grocery store. The clay is perfect for a variety of projects: holiday ornaments, jewelry or for press molds. The clay will harden completely by air-drying with a bright white finish. For the holidays you can roll the hardened piece in cinnamon for an old-time effect.

Ingredients:
1 cup water
1 cup salt
1 cup cornstarch

1) Mix 1 cup water and 1 cup cornstarch. 2) Heat in a saucepan over medium heat until the mixture thickens. 3) Add 1 cup salt. 4) Stir together in the saucepan until the mixture forms a firm ball. 5) Remove from the stove and allow to cool. 6) Use immediately or store the clay in a sealed plastic bag.

The clay can be flattened or rolled into shapes, and then air-dried for several days until rock-hard. For immediate results, bake the clay in a conventional oven at 250 degrees for 15 minutes. After the clay has hardened, it may be painted and decorated for use as jewelry or ornaments.

Paint

This recipe is great for low functioning adults or children who might want to sample the paint. It's also a great option if you haven't got time to get to the craft store or don't have a budget that will allow you to purchase expensive supplies. You can mix this up in your kitchen in about 5-10 minutes, and it will store up to 2 months in the refrigerator. I recommend using clean, recycled ketchup bottles or Tupperware containers for storage.

208

The consistency is good and the pigment will rival any commercial product out there.

Ingredients:
1 cup cornstarch
2 cups water
¼ cup food coloring
¼ cup liquid dish soap

1) Combine the cornstarch and the water in a saucepan. 2) Stir over medium heat until the mixture thickens. 3) Remove from the stove. 4) Add the food coloring (one color per batch). 5) Beat until the paint reaches a smooth consistency. 6) Add the liquid dish soap and beat again until completely homogenous. If the mixture is too thick, add more water as needed—a little at a time. Store in a plastic container in the refrigerator for up to 2 months.

8. Prescription Medications for Alzheimer 's Disease

Several prescription drugs are approved by the U.S. Food and Drug Administration (FDA) to treat people who have been diagnosed with Alzheimer's disease. There are many still in the pipeline with ongoing research and drug trials. It is important to understand that none of these medications stops the disease itself. I included this in the appendix as changes are frequent and you need to check with your doctor what is currently available.

Treatment for Mild to Moderate AD

Medications called cholinesterase inhibitors are prescribed for mild to moderate Alzheimer's disease. These drugs may help delay or prevent symptoms from becoming worse for a limited time and may help control some behavioral symptoms. The medications include: Razadyne® (galantamine), previously known as Reminyl®, Exelon® (rivastigmine), Aricept® (donepezil) and Cognex® (tacrine). Cognex® is no longer actively marketed by the manufacturer. Scientists do not yet fully understand how cholinesterase inhibitors work to treat Alzheimer's disease, but current research indicates that they prevent the breakdown of acetylcholine, a brain chemical believed to be important for memory and thinking. As the disease progresses, the brain produces less and less acetylcholine; therefore, cholinesterase inhibitors may eventually lose their effect.

No published study directly compares these drugs at this time. Because they work in a similar way, it is not expected that switching from one of these drugs to another will produce significantly different results. However, an Alzheimer's patient may respond better to one drug than another.

Treatment for Moderate to Severe AD

A medication known as Namenda® (memantine) is an N-methyl D-aspartate (NMDA) antagonist and is prescribed for the treatment of moderate to severe Alzheimer's disease. Studies have shown that the main effect of Namenda® is to delay progression of some of the symptoms of moderate to severe Alzheimer's disease. The medication may allow patients to maintain certain daily functions a little longer. The activities of daily living like dressing, bathing or using the bathroom alone may be preserved for a bit longer on such medications. Namenda® is believed to work by regulating glutamate, another important brain chemical that, when produced in excessive amounts, may lead to brain cell death. Because NMDA antagonists work very differently from cholinesterase inhibitors, the two types of drugs can be prescribed in combination. The FDA has also approved Aricept® for the treatment of moderate to severe Alzheimer's disease. These drugs can be used with other non pharmacological treatments aimed at slowing down the disease.

Dosage and Side Effects

Usually patients are started at low doses and gradually the dose is increased based on how well a patient tolerates the drug. There is some evidence that certain patients may benefit from higher doses of the cholinesterase inhibitor medications. The higher the dose, the more likely are side effects. Your prescribing doctor will be aware of the side affects and a list of them will be available from your pharmacist.

Patients may be drug-sensitive in other ways. Usually a patient is taking more than one medication and interactions can occur. Patients should be monitored when any new drug is started. Report any unusual symptoms to your doctor right away. It is important to follow the doctor's instructions when taking any medication, including additional vitamins and herbal or nutritional supplements and other over the counter medications and supplements. Also, let the doctor know before adding or changing any medications.

One example of side effects in the use of cholinesterase inhibitors is that it can increase risk of stomach ulcers, and because prolonged use of non-steroidal anti-inflammatory drugs (NSAIDs) such as aspirin or ibuprofen can also cause stomach ulcers, NSAIDs should be used with caution in combination with these medications. Many older people suffer from arthritis and simple aches and pains. We commonly use these NSAIDS and because they are over the counter often forget to mention them to our doctor. Cold remedies are other medications that can cause serious side effects so remember to consider any pill or liquid or cream that you use for any "remedy" when speaking with your doctor.

Works Cited

"ABC News: Readers Respond: Plight of Caring for Aging Parents Touched Many." ABC News: Online news, breaking news, feature stories and more. 23 June 2007 <http://abcnews.go.com/Health/ElderCare/story?id=3330502&page=1>.

Abraham, Ruth. When Words Have Lost Their Meaning: Alzheimer's Patients Communicate through Art. Westport, CT: Praeger Publishers, 2004.

Addington-Hall, J, and L Kalra. "Who should measure quality of life?" BMJ 322.7299 (2001): 1417-1420.

Aldridge, David. Music Therapy In Dementia Care. London: Jessica Kingsley, 2000.

Aldridge, David. Music Therapy Research & Practice In Medicine: From Out of the Silence. London: Jessica Kingsley, 1996.

"Alzheimer Care: Ethical Guidelines, Intimacy and Sexuality." Alzheimer Society of Canada . 2 Nov. 2007 <http://www.alzheimer.ca/english/care/ethics-intimacy.htm>.

"Alzheimer's Association Home." Alzheimer's Association Home. 11 Oct. 2007 <http://alz.org>.

"Alzheimer's Disease Research Foundation ." Alzheimer's Disease Research Foundation . 7 July 2007 <http://www.alzheimers-

research.org/currentresearch.htm>.

"Alzheimer's Foundation of America." Alzheimer's Foundation of America. 11 Oct. 2007 <http://www.alzfdn.org>.

"Alzheimer's Home." NIA Home. 11 Oct. 2007 <http://www.nia.nih.gov/alzheimers>.

Areosa Sastre, A, R Mcshane, and N Minakaran. "Memantine for dementia.." Cochrane Database Syst Review 0.1 (2008): 0. http://www.cochrane.org/reviews/en/ab003154.ht ml. null. null. 23 Mar. 2008.

Association, Hospice & Palliative Nurses. Core Curriculum for the Generalist Hospice and Palliative Nurse. Dubuque, Iowa: Kendall/Hunt Publishing company, 2005.

Ballard, Edna , and C Poer. Sexuality and the Alzheimer's Patient. Durham, North Carolina: Duke University Press, 1993.

Barnes, Mary-Michola, Barry M. Cohen, and Anita B. Rankin. Managing Traumatic Stress Through Art: Drawing from the Center. Baltimore: Sidran Press, 1995.

Barrett, Anna , and Kevin Scott. "Dementia Syndromes: Evaluation and Treatment." expert review of neurotherapies 7.4 (2007): 407-422.

Barry, Fanny. I Wish I Knew Series. Boston: That Barry Girl Partnership, 2005.

Beckett, Laurel, Clifford R Jack, William Jagust, Susanne G Mueller, Ronald C Petersen, Leon J Thal, Arthur W Toga, John Q Trojanowski, and Michael W Weiner.

"Ways toward an early diagnosis in Alzheimer's disease: The Alzheimer's Disease Neuroimaging Initiative (ADNI)." Alzheimers Dement 1.1 (2005): 55-66.

Bennett, P.D., L.M.T. Byrne-Davis, and G.K. Wilcock. "How are Quality of Life Ratings Made? Toward a Model of Quality of Life in People with Dementia." Quality of Life Research 15.5 (2006): 855-865.

Bjoro, K, and K Herr. "Tools for Assessment of Pain in Nonverbal Older Adults with Dementia: A State-of-the-Science Review." Journal of Pain and Symptom Management 31.2 (2000): 170-192.

Blakemore, Bill. "ABC News: Art Awakens Alzheimer's Patients' Minds." ABC News: Online news, breaking news, feature stories and more. 2 Nov. 2007 <http://abcnews.go.com/WNT/Health/story?id=21 46253>.

Brotons, Melissa, and Susan Koger. "The impact of music therapy on language functioning in dementia." Journal of Music Therapy 37.3 (2000): 183-195.

Calkins, M, S Slaughter, and M Eliasziw. "Measuring Physical and Social Environments in Nursing Homes for People with Middle to Late-Stage Dementia." Journal of the American Geriatrics Society 54.9 (2006): 1436-1441.

Camp, Cameron J. Montessori Based Activities for Persons, Vol.II. Beachwood, Ohio: Menorah Park Center For Senior Living, 2006.

Camp, Cameron J. Montessori-Based Activities for Persons With Dementia Vol. 1. Baltimore: Health Professions Press, 1999.

Celia, Lisa, and Jackie Nasso. Dementia Care: InService Training Modules for Long-Term Care. Forence, KY: Thomson Delmar Learning, 2006.

Chavin, Melanie. "Music as Communication." Journal of Music Therapy 34.3 (1997): 165-186.

"Choosing Senior Housing and Residential Care." Help guide: A trusted non-profit resource for mental health, healthy lifestyles and aging issues. 12 Mar. 2008 <http://www.helpguide.org/elder/senior_housing_residential_care_types.htm>.

Clare, Linda, and Pam Shakespeare. "Negotiating the Impact of Forgetting: Dimensions of Resistance in Task-Oriented Conversations between People with Early-Stage Dementia and their Partners." Dementia 3.2 (2004): 211-232.

Clarke, Charlotte. "Family care-giving for people with dementia: some implications for policy and professional practice." Journal of Advanced Nursing 29.3 (2007): 712-720. 6 July 2007 <http://www.blackwell-synergy.com/doi/abs/10.1046/j.1365-2648.1999.00940.x>.

Coste, Joanne Koenig. Learning to Speak Alzheimer's: A Groundbreaking Approach for Everyone Dealing with the Disease. Boston: Houghton Mifflin, 2004.

Cummings, Jeffrey L., and Mario Mendez. Dementia: A Clinical Approach. St. Louis, Missouri: Butterworth-Heinemann, 2003.

Cummins, R.A.. "Moving from the quality of life concept to a theory." Journal of Intellectual Disability Research 49.10 (2005): 699-706. 23 Mar. 2008

<http://www.blackwell-synergy.com/doi/abs/10.1111/j.1365-2788.2005.00738.x>.

Davis, William B, Kate E Gfeller, and Michael H Thaut. An Introduction To Music Therapy: Theory and Practice. New York City, NY: McGraw-Hill, 1998.

"Dementia: Not always Alzheimer's." CNN.com—Breaking News, U.S., World, Weather, Entertainment & Video News. 23 Aug. 2007 <http://www.cnn.com/HEALTH/library/AZ/0000 3.html>.

"Dementia: Not always Alzheimer's." CNN.com—Breaking News, U.S., World, Weather, Entertainment & Video News. 23 Mar. 2008 <http://www.cnn.com/HEALTH/library/AZ/0000 3.html>.

Droes, Rose-Marie, Jacomine Lange, Gideon Mellenbergh, and Miel Ribbe. "Quality of life in dementia in perspective; an explorative study of variations in opinions among people with dementia and their professional caregivers, and in literature." Dementia: the International Journal of Social Research and Practice 5.4 (2006): 533-558. 23 May 2007 <http://www.scie-socialcareonline.org.uk/profile.asp?guid=43a948e5 -3290-43df-b735-f83939553dae>.

Erikson, Erik H.. Psychological Issues (Identity and the Life Cycle, Volume 1). New York: International Universities Press, 1980.

Field, Tiffany. Massage Therapy Research. Philadelphia, PA: Churchill Livingstone, 2006.

Field, Tiffany. Touch Therapy. Philadelphia, PA: Churchill

Livingstone, 2000.

Geldmacher, D, and P Whitehouse. "Differential diagnosis of Alzheimer's disease.." Neurology 48.5 Suppl 6 (1997): null.

Goleman, Daniel. Emotional Intelligence: 10th Anniversary Edition; Why It Can Matter More Than IQ. New York City, NY: Bantam, 2006.

Hanser, Suzanne B. The New MusicTherapist's Handbook. Boston: Berklee Press Publications, 2000.

Heikki, Ikaheimo, and A Laitinen. "Dimensions of Personhood." Journal of Consciousness Studies 14.5-6 (2007): 6-16.

Innes, Anthea, and Louise Mc Cabe. Evaluation in Dementia Care. London: Jessica Kingsley Publishers, 2006.

Innes, Anthea. Healing Arts Therapies and Person-Centered Dementia Care (Bradford Dementia Group). London: Jessica Kingsley Publishers, 2001.

Kennedy, Randy. "BrainBlog: Art Therapy in Dementia." BrainBlog. 31 Oct. 2005. 2 Nov. 2007 <http://neuropsychological.blogspot.com/2005/10 /art-therapy-in-dementia.html>.

Kimble, Melvin. Aging, Spirituality, and Religion: A Handbook (Aging, Spirituality, and Religion). Minneapolis: Augsburg Fortress Publishers, 2004.

Kinney, J.M., and C.A. Rentz. "Observed well-being Among Individuals with Dementia: Memories in the Making: an Art Program, versus Other Structured Activity." American Journal of Alzheimer'€™s Disease and Other Dementias 20.4 (2005): 220-7.

Kitwood, Tom. <u>Dementia Reconsidered: the Person Comes First</u>. Buckingham: Open University Press, 1997.

Kramer, E. "The Art Therapistâ€™s Third Hand." <u>American Journal of Art Therapy</u> 24 (1986): 71-86.

Kumamoto, Keigo, Masakazu Washio, and Yumiko Arai. "Assessment of family caregiver burden in the context of the LTC insurance system." <u>Geriatrics & Gerontology International</u> S1 (2004): S53â€"S55.

Kydd, P. "Using music therapy to help a client with Alzheimer's Disease adapt to long-term care." <u>American Journal of Alzheimer's Disease and Other Dementias</u> 16(2).March-April 2001 (2001): 103-108.

"Learn More About Massage and the Benefits." <u>Massage Therapy Information, Find a Massage Therapist, Careers In Massage, Massage Schools, Massage State Regulations, Bodywork Glossary, and More Available.</u>. 23 Aug. 2007 <http://www.massagetherapy.com/learnmore/ben efits.php>.

"Life Extension Foundation—Highest Quality Vitamins And Supplements." <u>Life Extension Foundation—Highest Quality Vitamins And Supplements</u>. 11 Oct. 2007 <http://www.lef.org>.

Lyketsos, Constantine G., Peter V. Rabins, and Cynthia D. Steele. <u>Practical Dementia Care</u>. New York: Oxford University Press, USA, 2006.

Mc Clane, Kenneth A. <u>Driving.(Family)(Alzheimer's disease patients): An article from: The Antioch Review</u>. Chicago: Thomson Gale, 2006.

Omelan, C. "Approach to managing behavioural disturbances in dementia." Can Fam Physician 52.null (2006): 191-199.

Pereira, J, S Raffin, and S Sinclair. "A thematic review of the spirituality literature within palliative care.." J Palliat Med 9.2 (2006): 464-479.

Pollack, Andrew. "Scientists Report Advances in Diagnosing Alzheimer's Disease Years Before Onset." New York Times 15 Oct. 2007. 15 Oct. 2007 <nytimes.com>.

Purtilo, Ruth B. Ethical Foundations of Palliative Care for Alzheimer Disease. Baltimore: The Johns Hopkins University Press, 2004.

Rockwood, K. "Mixed dementia: Alzheimer's and cerebrovascular disease." Int Psychogeriatr 15 Suppl 1.null (2003): 39-46.

Singer, T. "Want to Know What Makes a Creative Genius Tick? Neuroscience Gives Us Some Clues." Inc Magazine 0.September (2002): 1-3. 20 Nov. 2007 <www.inc.com>.

Spooren, W. "Research watch: Spoken and written, verbal and nonverbal communication." Document Design 4.3 (2003): 272-274.

Swaminathan, Dr. Rajesh V.. "ABC News: Study: Alzheimer's Medications Help, but Just a Little." ABC News: Online news, breaking news, feature stories and more. 2 Nov. 2007 <http://abcnews.go.com/Health/story?id=1537258 >.

"University of Sussex Media Release 15th January 1999New Research Makes the Link Between Arts and Minds."

University of Sussex Homepage. 15 Jan. 1999. 2 Nov. 2007 <http://www.sussex.ac.uk/press_office/media/media44.html>.

Vandecreek, Larry. Spiritual Care for Persons With Dementia: Fundamentals for Pastoral Practice. New York : Haworth Press, 2001.

Vanderbilt, Shirley. "Massage Therapy Massage Bodywork Massage Therapy Schools Massage Therapy Career." Massage Therapy Massage Bodywork Massage Therapy Schools Massage Therapy Career with MassageTherapy.com. 2 Nov. 2007 <http://www.massagetherapy.com>.

Vicioso, B.A. "Dementia: When is it not Alzheimer disease?." American Journal of the Medical Sciences 324.2 (2002): 84-95.

Volicer, L. Enhancing the Quality of Life in Advanced Dementia. New York: Routledge, 1999.

Warren, Mary Anne. Moral Status: Obligations to Persons and Other Living Things (Issues in Biomedical Ethics). New York: Oxford University Press, USA, 2000.

Weiner, Myron. "The quality of life in late-stage dementia (Qualid) Scale." J Am Med Dir Assn 1 (2000): 114-116.

Index

Printed in the United States
121522LV00002B/115-117/P